B

A Straight Forward
and Excellence in M

C000171377

First Edition

Author: Rob Schwarz, MSc, RN

Rob Schwarz has worked in the health environment for
many years and is currently a nurse practitioner in practice
in large London teaching hospital.

Editor: Andrew Le Grove
BSc (Hons), PG Cert, RN

Andrew Le Grove has also worked in the health
environment for many years and is currently a nurse
practitioner in practice in large London teaching hospital.

Sub editor: Patrick Stork

This book is produced by the publishing house of Essential
Knowledge Ltd in collaboration with A&A Training Ltd.

Essential
Knowledge
□ ■ ■Limited

Publishing, Consultancy, Conferencing
Rochester, United Kingdom

Published in April 2006 by

ESSENTIAL KNOWLEDGE LIMITED
PO Box 415
Rochester
Kent
ME2 3WP

www.eskn.co.uk
0870 760 1309

First Edition

British Library Cataloguing in Publication Data

A catalogue record for this book is available from the
British Library

ISBN 0-9552910-03
ISBN 978-0-9552910-0-5

Printed and bound in Great Britain by:
TT Litho, Rochester, Kent.

Contents

Contents

Acknowledgements

This book is dedicated to my wife Caryl, without her
support and kind patience it would not have
been possible.

The support, motivation and enthusiasm of my friend and
editor, Andy Le Grove, has been immeasurable in the
creation of this book.

Preface to the first edition

The experience of most staff in the NHS is one of having to often work in ways that are new to them, and in ways that their professional training did not equip to them deal with.

The writing of this book is in response to the widening role of many professionals not just in the clinical arena, but in many other endeavours such as management within the hospital at night project, bed management, management of violence and aggression and ethical issues, for example.

This book is intended primarily for clinicians such as nurses, nurse practitioners, student nurses, operational managers, midwives and healthcare assistants who work in association with medicine and who are experiencing role expansion.

This book is best used is by the clinician at the bedside who may need the reassurance of the key information within its text and can easily be carried to the bedside in the uniform pocket.

The purpose and aspiration of this, the first in a series of books, is to enable and underpin the clinician in whatever environment they find themselves in.

DISCLAIMER

The drug information presented in this book was compiled from published reference sources and pharmaceutical package inserts. Every effort has been made to ensure that the dosage regimens presented are accurate at the time of publication. All other care and guidelines have been checked to ensure accuracy.

As a result of ongoing research, clinical experience, and changes in recognised guidelines and legislation, the author and editors ask that the reader not use this book as the sole source of any care provided, or drugs administered.

The author, editors and publisher, cannot be responsible for any liability, loss, injury, or damage incurred as a consequence, directly or indirectly, from the use and application of any of the contents of this book. The ultimate responsibility lies with the healthcare professional on the basis of their professional license, registration, experience, and knowledge of the patient, to determine the correct care or drugs, and overall best course of action for the patient.

The patient in peri-arrest, or in respiratory or cardiac arrest

In this chapter the sick patient is defined in the most extreme and urgent of situations, that is, the cardiac arrest.

The clinician is guided through a simple yet detailed structure of how to respond to the cardiac arrest when they are the first member of the team on hand.

The patient is also presented in the near arrest, or peri-arrest, situation and the clinician is guided through first level assessment and key interventions to be delivered at this time.

The chapter develops with an in depth look at the advanced management of the cardiac arrest with an exploration of the ALS algorithm.

Chapter 1 Contents

Chapter 1 Contents

First-glance assessment of the sick patient

When initially assessing a patient who has been highlighted to you as somebody that has rapidly deteriorated, your assessment should be structured along the following lines:

- Is this patient likely to arrest imminently?

- How long can I spend assessing before acting?

- What signs can be ascertained immediately?

- What other information is available now?

- What more information can be obtained?

Do I put out a crash call?

Your crash call number (Cardiac Arrest / Emergency)

Remember, it is OK to put out a crash call even though the patient has not as yet had a respiratory or cardiac arrest.

The resuscitation of a peri-arrest patient invariably has a better outcome than the resuscitation of an arrested patient.

This is that information that you can get at the bedside. It is the information that will enable your first assessment priority "Is an arrest imminent?"

Are there signs of low cardiac output?

- Sweaty

- Pallor

- Centrally cold or cold extremities

- Clammy

- Impaired consciousness

Are there signs of respiratory distress?

- Breathlessness – can the patient speak in full sentences?

- Cyanosis

- Poor chest movement

- Agonal breathing

- Tachypnoea

- Exhaustion and confusion

M.O.V.E

First line emergency manoeuvres for the practitioner in the healthcare setting

When you arrive at the scene of an acutely deteriorated or peri-arrest patient within the healthcare environment, there are a number of actions that can be taken which will be of immediate benefit in second stage assessment and preparation for further deterioration if the patient proceeds to respiratory or cardiac arrest.

These actions, once embedded in the nurse's practice, can reduce anxiety, speed up management, assist the direction of others and ultimately may improve patient out come.

M = Monitor: Attach the patient to a cardiac monitor. If the patient collapses at this stage with no cardiac output, a greater range of management options are available to you, see VT/VF management under Chapter 3. Acquire and monitor vital observations, blood pressure, heart rate, oxygen saturations and respiratory rate.

O = Oxygen: Oxygen is indicated in most peri-arrest situations. Administer high flow oxygen. Caution should be given to patients who have, or are known to have, high arterial blood carbon dioxide levels. However, in life threatening hypoxia high flow oxygen is still given.

V = Venous access: A peri-arrest patient will need intravenous intervention of some kind and if the patient proceeds to cardiac arrest this procedure becomes more difficult. See Cannulation and venepuncture under Chapter 4.

E = ECG and Expert Help: A 12-lead electrocardiogram (ECG) is particularly useful in this situation if the collapse is a cardiac mediated event. The ECG can give valuable information about other problems such as electrolyte imbalance, see interpreting under Chapter 3. **Expert help must be summoned.** This may be by calling a medical emergency team, Cardiac Arrest team, or by fast bleeping a specific team member such as the anaesthetist or medical registrar.

First response in the suspected arrest

Ensure your own safety

In the hospital or healthcare environment this will include observance of universal precautions, including wearing gloves, considering additional barrier precautions if infection threat is evident, see universal precautions under Chapter 16.

Assessment

Open airway with a head tilt, chin lift or jaw thrust (if the cervical spine is at risk of damage).

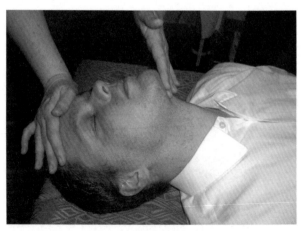

Look, listen and feel

Assess the patient's breathing by getting close to their mouth and **looking** across their chest for signs of movement. **Listen** for breath sounds at the same time and **feel** for the movement of air from breathing upon your cheek.

The trained healthcare professional should concurrently palpate the carotid artery to assess whether or not the patient has a beating heart.

Do not delay resuscitation whilst trying to locate a carotid pulse.

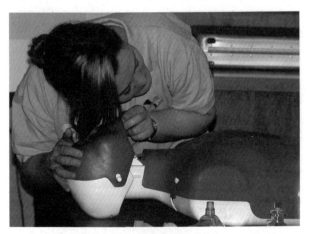

Jaw thrust

If the reason for the patient's collapse is unclear or if the collapse is to the floor, consider the mechanism of collapse or injury. If your patient has damaged their cervical spine in the process of a fall then the way you approach them and the way in which you open the airway may have a profound influence on the outcome.

The head tilt chin lift as described in the universal algorithm is contra indicated in cervical lesions as this manoeuvre can transect the spinal chord if the cervical vertebra is unstable. In this instance the recommended approach is to open the airway with the jaw thrust.

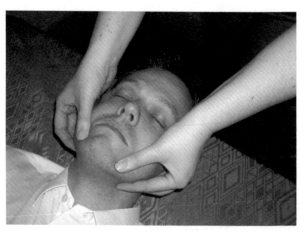

The jaw thrust opens the airway by pushing the jaw forward and applying pressure with the fingers at the angulations of the mandible with a counter press applied by the thumbs in the region of the zygoma.

This manoeuvre forces the tongue away from the airway whilst keeping the cervical spine in alignment.

Summon help. In the healthcare environment this will be the crash call and defibrillator.

Where there is no circulation, chest compressions should be started at a ratio of 30 compressions to 2 breaths in the adult patient.

Following chest compressions, you should give 2 effective ventilation breaths. Each breath should take one second. Do not wait for the chest to fall before resuming chest compressions.

Chest compressions

The anatomical marker for hand position is the centre of the chest, avoiding the xiphisternum.

Do not delay chest compressions by using complex methods to locate the position for your hands on the victim's chest.

Keeping your arms straight, moving from your hips commence the compressions at a rate of 100 per minute.

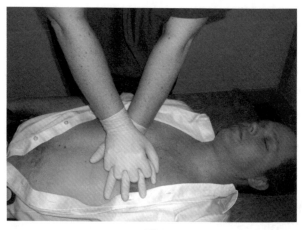

The rescue breaths

If appropriate in terms of algorithm, give rescue breaths:

- Open airway – Head tilt, chin lift. Contraindicated in cervical spine injury.

- Pinch nose.

- Examine mucous membrane for lesions, cuts or any breech of integrity as there is a risk of blood borne infection.

- Take a deep breath. Make a mouth to mouth seal and blow into the victim's mouth.

- Watch the chest rise from the corner of your eye.

- Take no longer than one second per breath.

BLS algorithm

Resuscitation Council (UK) 2005

Adult Basic Life Support

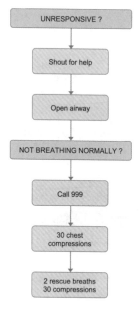

Chest compressions begin first at a rate of 30 compressions to 2 breaths.

Cardiac arrest

There are in effect 3 kinds of cardiac arrest, they are:

- Ventricular fibrillation (VF) and pulseless Ventricular tachycardia (VT) are known as shockable rhythms

- Pulseless electrical activity (PEA) – Non shockable rhythm

- Asystole – Non shockable rhythm

VF and pulseless VT are cardiac rhythms that cause a cessation of cardiac output and are therefore terminal.

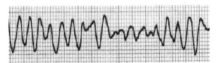

Ventricular fibrillation

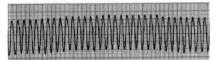

Ventricular tachycardia

Defibrillation algorithm

Resuscitation Council (UK) 2005

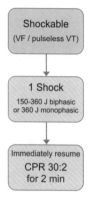

Within the 2005 resuscitation guidelines, there has been a new approach to defibrillation. The guidelines reflect research findings that demonstrate greater efficiency of defibrillation when the myocardium has been oxygenated.

In practice, this means that there are no stacks of defibrillation but only one. If this is ineffective there should be a resumption of CPR for a further two minutes, prior to the next shock.

The nature of defibrillation

Electrical defibrillation is well established as the only effective therapy for cardiac arrest due to VF or pulseless VT.

Restoration of effective ventricular contraction is paramount in this situation as cerebral hypoxia injury will begin after 3 minutes, less if there was a period of hypoxia prior to the arrest.

The only successful management is prompt recognition of these rhythms and equally prompt defibrillation.

Defibrillation is the depolarisation of a critical mass of myocardium simultaneously to a restoration of the natural pace making function within the heart muscle tissue.

In many environments an Automated External Defibrillator (AED) is the defibrillator of choice, this equipment has the advantage of:

- Ease of use as there are verbal prompts throughout deployment.

- Safety as it uses hands free pads rather than paddles.

- Biphasic wave form which delivers lower energy to the myocardium thereby causing less damage. Biphasic defibrillators have first shock efficiency of up to 90% and are significantly more efficient than mono-phasic defibrillators.

AED algorithm

Resuscitation Council (UK) 2005

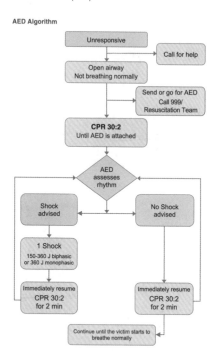

AED Algorithm

Unresponsive

Call for help

Open airway
Not breathing normally

Send or go for AED
Call 999/
Resuscitation Team

CPR 30:2
Until AED is attached

AED
assesses
rhythm

Shock
advised

No Shock
advised

1 Shock
150-360 J biphasic
or 360 J monophasic

Immediately resume
CPR 30:2
for 2 min

Immediately resume
CPR 30:2
for 2 min

Continue until the victim starts to
breathe normally

Using a manual defibrillator or AED safely

If shock advised (AED prompt) or you establish the patient needs defibrillation, you are responsible for the safety of everyone present when using the defibrillator.

- Assess the patient

- Apply paddles or pads, if appropriate

- Ensure everybody stands clear of the victim

- Shout "*Oxygen away*"

- State "*Charging paddles on chest stand clear*"

- Check the **head** end of the victim is clear

- Check the **middle** area of the victim is clear

- Check the **feet** end of the victim is clear

- Check **you** are clear

- Ensure the victim is still in VF/VT by checking the monitor, if available, immediately before delivering the shock

- Deliver shock

ALS algorithm

The approach to resuscitation has achieved an industry standard within the fields of medical, nursing and professions allied to medicine. This has been achieved essentially through the structure of the Resuscitation Council, which has in turn given a strategic format to the acquisition and deployment of best practice.

Fundamental to the implementation of resuscitation guidelines is an approach that is consistent, prioritises key interventions, enables and empowers individuals, and enables a team approach.

A core element of the Resuscitation Council approach is the management structure that is described, taught and acted on in the clinical environment and the adherence to a succinct and direct diagrammatic instruction in the format of the algorithm.

ALS algorithm

Resuscitation Council (UK) 2005

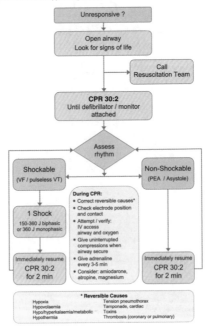

Adult Advanced Life Support Algorithm

Non-shockable rhythms: Asystole and pulseless electrical activity

- Give CPR (2 minute intervals)

- Give epinephrine (Adrenaline 1mg)

- Repeat at 3 to 5 minute intervals

- Secure access

- Secure airway and oxygen therapy

- Atropine 3mg can be given

- Consider pacing if indicated

- Treat the causes

Epinephrine (Adrenaline) can be given via an ET tube if vascular access proves a problem, in which case double the dose and ventilate the lungs 5 times following administration to disperse the drug.

Atropine can also be given via this route, and double the dose to 6 mg.

When giving drugs via a peripheral vein they should be followed by a flush of 20ml normal saline, to ensure the drugs are pushed towards the heart.

Drugs in cardiac arrest

Epinephrine (Adrenaline) 1 mg has the effect of vasoconstriction, which causes stimulation of alpha receptors, which increases myocardial and cerebral perfusion pressure.

Atropine 3mg is given to provide a blockade of the vagal nerve. This is a one off 3mg dose, further doses are ineffective. Atropine should be given in asystole and in PEA where the monitored rhythm is consistent with a Bradycardia (heart rate less than 60bpm).

Bicarbonate 50mmols should be used to correct acidosis in, or after, the arrest situation where the arterial blood gas shows a pH of less than 7.1, or if the cardiac arrest is associated with tricyclic overdose or hyperkalaemia.

Amiodarone 300mg made up to 20ml with dextrose 5% can be given to treat cardiac arrest due to VF or pulseless VT, following 3 unsuccessful attempts at defibrillation. A further dose of 150mg can be considered in shock-refractory VF/VT.

Calcium Chloride / Calcium Gluconate 10ml of 10% can be given to treat Hyperkalaemia, Hypocalcaemia, Calcium channel blockers overdose, and an overdose of magnesium.

Reversible causes of cardiac arrest

The 4 Hs and the 4 Ts

- Hypoxia

- Hypovolaemia

- Hyperkalaemia/Hypocalcaemia

- Hypothermia

- Tension pneumothorax

- Tamponade

- Therapeutic or toxic substance

- Thrombo-embolic or mechanical circulatory obstruction

Hypoxia – give 100% oxygen therapy.

Hypovolaemia – secure good access and given large volumes of appropriate fluids.

Hyperkalaemia / Hypocalcaemia – use blood tests, ECG and patient history to ascertain the likely hood of these causes.

Hypothermia – should be suspected in submersion or immersion injuries. Manage by warming the patient and remember that hypothermia protects the victim's brain tissue and therefore death can only be declared once the patient is warm.

Tension pneumothorax – diagnosed by percussion of a hyper resonate chest on the affected side with a deviated trachea. In the arrest situation you should decompress with by needle thoracentsis.

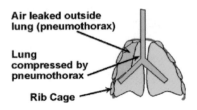

Air leaked outside lung (pneumothorax)

Lung compressed by pneumothorax

Rib Cage

Initially a brown or orange intravenous cannula (Gauge 14) should be inserted in the second intercostal space, followed by a chest drain, when an experienced practitioner is available to insert one.

This diagnosis should be highly suspected if the arrest followed the insertion of a central venous catheter.

Cardiac **tamponade** is the accumulation of blood or other fluid into the pericardial sac, when this happens acutely, and significantly, it can lead to PEA.

Diagnosis of cardiac tamponade is made when there are distended neck veins, high central venous pressure and hypotension, although in the arrest situation this information is not necessarily available. When there is a history of a penetrating chest wound this diagnosis should be considered. Management is with a needle pericarsdiocentesis.

Therapeutic or toxic substances may well be the likely cause of the arrest but can often only be established after a blood test, at which time antidote (if available) can be given, until that time the management is supportive.

Thromboembolic or mechanical circulatory obstruction is most commonly massive pulmonary emboli and the management for this is vigorous chest compression in the first instance, other options are thrombolysis, cardiopulmonary bypass or surgical removal of the clot.

Peri arrest arrhythmias algorithm

Having established that you have a very sick patient on your hands you have to move quickly and identify:

- Is the problem related to an arrhythmia?

- If so, what is it?

- What is the first line management?

The following signs are significant in the peri arrest scenario:

- Signs of low cardiac output

- Increased sympathetic activity – the body is optimising core circulation at the expense of the peripheries

- Pallor

- Sweating

- Cold

- Clammy

- Cold extremities

- Lowered cerebral blood flow, resulting in:

    - Impaired consciousness

    - Confusion

    - Unconsciousness

Excessive tachycardia

In excessive tachycardia the diastolic blood pressure is less well maintained, diastolic being the point at which coronary blood flow is achieved, therefore the patient is at high risk of myocardial ischemia.

This phenomena occurs at a different rate in broad complex tachycardia (>150 beats per minute) than narrow complex tachycardia (>200 beats per minute) as the body tolerates broad complex tachycardia less well.

Excessive bradycardia

This is defined as less than 60 beats per minute, although a vulnerable patient with low cardiac reserve may well be symptomatic at a higher rate.

Bradycardia algorithm

Resuscitation Council (UK) 2005

Bradycardia Algorithm
(includes rates inappropriately slow for haemodynamic state)

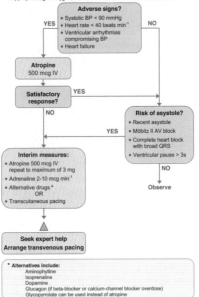

If appropriate, give oxygen, cannulate a vein, and record a 12-lead ECG

Adverse signs?
- Systolic BP < 90 mmHg
- Heart rate < 40 beats min⁻¹
- Ventricular arrhythmias compromising BP
- Heart failure

YES → **Atropine** 500 mcg IV

Satisfactory response?

YES

NO

Risk of asystole?
- Recent asystole
- Möbitz II AV block
- Complete heart block with broad QRS
- Ventricular pause > 3s

YES

NO → Observe

Interim measures:
- Atropine 500 mcg IV repeat to maximum of 3 mg
- Adrenaline 2-10 mcg min⁻¹
- Alternative drugs *
  OR
- Transcutaneous pacing

Seek expert help
Arrange transvenous pacing

* Alternatives include:
Aminophylline
Isoprenaline
Dopamine
Glucagon (if beta-blocker or calcium-channel blocker overdose)
Glycopyrrolate can be used instead of atropine

Tachycardia algorithm

Resuscitation Council (UK) 2005

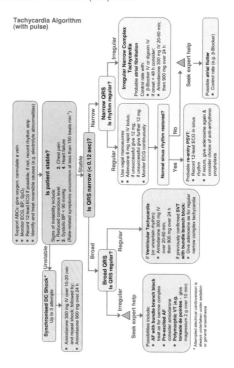

Tachycardia Algorithm
(with pulse)

Support ABCs: give oxygen; cannulate a vein
- Monitor ECG, BP, SpO₂
- Record 12-lead ECG if possible; if not, record rhythm strip
- Identify and treat reversible causes (e.g. electrolyte abnormalities)

Is patient stable?
Signs of instability include:
1. Reduced conscious level
2. Chest pain
3. Systolic BP < 90 mmHg
4. Heart failure
(Rate-related symptoms uncommon at less than 150 beats min⁻¹)

Unstable

Synchronised DC Shock*
Up to 3 attempts

- Amiodarone 300 mg IV over 10–20 min and repeat shock; followed by:
- Amiodarone 900 mg over 24 h

Stable

Is QRS narrow (< 0.12 sec)?

Broad — Broad QRS Is QRS regular?

Narrow — Narrow QRS Is rhythm regular?

Broad QRS — Irregular
Seek expert help

Possibilities include:
- **AF with bundle branch block** treat as for narrow complex
- **Pre-excited AF** consider amiodarone
- **Polymorphic VT** (e.g. torsade de pointes - give magnesium 2 g over 10 min)

Broad QRS — Regular
If Ventricular Tachycardia (or uncertain rhythm):
- Amiodarone 300 mg IV over 20–60 min; then 900 mg over 24 h

If previously confirmed SVT **with bundle branch block:**
- Give adenosine as for regular narrow complex tachycardia

Narrow QRS — Regular
- Use vagal manoeuvres
- Adenosine 6 mg rapid IV bolus; if unsuccessful give 12 mg; if unsuccessful give further 12 mg; Monitor ECG continuously

Normal sinus rhythm restored?

Yes — Probable re-entry PSVT:
- Record 12-lead ECG in sinus rhythm
- If recurs, give adenosine again & consider choice of anti-arrhythmic prophylaxis

No — Seek expert help

Possible atrial flutter
- Control rate (e.g. β-Blocker)

Narrow QRS — Irregular
Irregular Narrow Complex Tachycardia
Probable atrial fibrillation
Control rate with:
- β-Blocker IV or digoxin IV
If onset < 48 h consider:
- Amiodarone 300 mg IV 20–60 min; then 900 mg over 24 h

Seek expert help

*Attempted electrical cardioversion is always undertaken under sedation or general anaesthesia

41

Chapter 1 – Further reading

Chapter 1 – Further reading

Resuscitation Council (UK 2005 Editorial Chair Jerry Nolan.	2005	Advanced Life Support – Fifth Edition, Resuscitation Council, London.
International Liaison Committee on Resuscitation. Part 4 Advanced Life Support 2005.	2005	International consensus on cardiopulmonary resuscitation and emergency cardiovascular care science treatment with recommendations. Resuscitation 2005:67:213-247.
Smith GB et al.	2002	ALERT – A multi professional training course in the care of the acutely ill adult patient. Resuscitation 2002:52:281-286.
International Liaison Committee on Resuscitation. Part 3 Defibrillation.	2005	International consensus on cardiopulmonary resuscitation and emergency cardiovascular care science treatment with recommendations. 67:203-211.
Jevon P.	2001	A matter of life or death. Nursing Times 97 (37) 32-34.

Chapter 2

Advanced assessment of the chest

In Chapter 2 and Chapter 3, the clinician will be guided in advanced assessment skills. The diagrammatic approach enables bedside decision making by allowing comparison. For example a normal chest x-ray is shown from which the clinician can make an informed comparative judgement.

Clinicians using this book will be enabled by a systematic approach to interpretation that is intended to underpin the initial development of new skills, with a framework of infra structure upon which the clinician can build new expertise and insights.

Whilst fundamental, it must be remembered that these skills sit within an array of approaches and other skills that together craft the process of clinical decision making.

The practice and use of these assessment skills will only be of value when deployed in the greater context of good history taking, rapport building, empathy and the exercise of tacit knowledge that a seasoned clinician will apply intuitively.

To be a good clinician one must act on what you know, validate what you can see and communicate it in a language of the recipient.

For nurses and professionals allied to medicine, this means carrying forward the sense of knowing, and furnishing it with the approaches and language of bioscience. This is especially important when dealing across professional boundaries and maintaining the skill for communication that fosters an empathetic approach to the patient.

The skills described in Chapter 2 give the clinician an opportunity to examine the patient hands on, with a stethoscope, whilst auscultating the chest, the ability to interpret chest x-rays and the sampling and evaluation of arterial blood gases. All three skills individually can give a key insight into many problems, but together the clinician can triangulate these approaches to find a definitive conclusion to their findings.

Chapter 2 Contents

Chapter 2 Contents

Procedure for taking arterial blood gases

Taking an arterial blood sample is a relatively simple procedure but it is often considered difficult, advanced and the preserve of doctors.

It may be that the mystic repute of this procedure is due to it being carried out commonly at times of a sudden deterioration in a patient's condition, nevertheless, it is a procedure that once mastered, is as easy as cannulation of a peripheral vein.

When one considers the anatomy of the artery compared to the vein we can quickly see how the nature of the artery can contribute to the ease of the procedure.

The artery wall contains more muscle fibres than a vein which means it will hold its shape and not collapse even when the intrinsic pressure of the blood falls.

Arteries sit at a deeper level in the tissue than veins and are therefore less mobile.

Arteries are filled with blood pumped directly from the heart.

The procedure

Check collateral circulation – Allen's Test

This test is performed to ensure that there is collateral arterial supply to the hand from ulna artery. The potential disruption of the radial artery could be disastrous in the known but uncommon instance of the radial artery being the only supply of blood to the hand.

To perform the Allen's test

Occlude the radial and ulna arteries by applying pressure to them with your finger tips. The hand slowly blanches as the blood supply is interrupted.

When blanching is noted, release the pressure on the ulna artery and the hand should become rapidly pink thereby asserting collateral circulation.

Take the patient's history to confirm if there is coagulopathy or if the patient is receiving anti-coagulant therapy. You may need to reconsider undertaking this procedure.

Similarly peripheral vascular disease is a contraindication. However, both have to be considered against the value of undertaking the procedure in terms of the patient's further management.

Locate the artery by palpation of the pulsatile vessel at the radial site.

Run your finger from side to side over the vessel, estimating the depth beneath the skin and the direction in which it travels.

- Use a hepparinsed ABG syringe.

- Prepare the radial site. Brachial and femoral may also be used.

- Locate the radial artery by palpation.

- Expel heparin from syringe.

- Aim the needle bevel up at 45 degree angle, aiming upstream and away from the hand.

- Fill the syringe to a minimum of 1ml, under artery pressure.

- Remove the syringe and apply pressure to puncture site.

ABG Hints and Tips

1. Spend a couple of minutes locating the artery and the exact position you will enter the skin. Timely assessment most often results in success on the first attempt, less pain for the patient and a quicker all round technique.

2. If you are unable to locate the artery once you have entered the skin, withdraw the needle towards the skin, then change the angle and re-advance. This will reduce the pain the patient suffers following repeated piercing of the skin, and will save using many ABG syringe packs.

3. If a small amount of blood is present in the syringe, but not enough, and you are unsuccessful in gaining more, even though you feel you are in the artery, you may have to withdraw and change arms, as occasionally the radial artery will go in to spasm at the site of entry and you will be unable to continue on that arm.

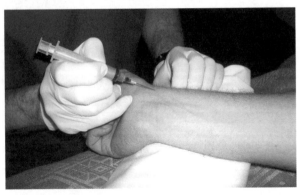

Normal ABG values

Normal Arterial Blood Gas values	
pH	7.35 to 7.45
PaO_2	10.8 to 15.0 kPa
$PaCO_2$	4.5 to 6.0 kPa
HCO_3	22 to 28 mmol/L
BE	+2 to -2 mmol/L

ABG interpretation

When interpreting arterial blood gases, you need to think of the nature of the measured chemicals identified in the ABG sample. If you know the characteristics of the chemicals measured, then you can anticipate what they will do.

Carbon Dioxide (CO_2) is a gas that is acidic in its nature – it will make a blood sample acidic if present in large quantities. A high CO_2 equals acidosis. The other thing to remember about CO_2 is that it is a by-product of breathing and if it is present in high quantities the cause is therefore respiratory.

Bicarbonate (HCO_3) is a chemical that mops up acid and the process of mopping up causes HCO_3 to be used up. Therefore, in acidosis

HCO_3 levels will fall and the reverse will happen in alkalosis, that is, HCO_3 will rise.

Acidosis occurs when the pH is below 7.35 and there are two types of acidosis:

- Respiratory where high levels of CO_2 are found.

- Metabolic where low levels of HCO_3 are found.

It follows that if there are two types of acidosis, then there will be two types of alkalosis. Again, these are defined by the level of CO_2 and HCO_3 present.

Alkalosis occurs when the pH is above 7.45 and the two types are:

- Respiratory where low levels of CO_2 are found.

- Metabolic where high levels of HCO_3 are found.

Compensation

The body will compensate for an abnormal pH which can change the ABG picture.

In respiratory acidosis the kidneys will attempt to compensate by retaining HCO_3 and therefore both CO_2 and HCO_3 will be elevated in respiratory acidosis with renal compensation.

Inversely, respiratory alkalosis with renal compensation will be seen as low CO_2 with low HCO_3 levels.

Respiratory compensation will occur in metabolic acidosis with the patients breathing at a greater rate in order to blow off the CO_2. Therefore metabolic acidosis with respiratory compensation will be seen as low HCO_3 with a low CO_2.

The inverse of this situation is a slower and shallower breathing pattern which results in the accumulation of the acid gas CO_2 as respiratory compensation to the metabolic alkalosis.

ABG interpretation table

Acid base disorder	pH	CO$_2$	HCO$_3$
Respiratory acidosis	↓	↑	N
Metabolic acidosis	↓	N	↓
Respiratory alkalosis	↑	↓	N
Metabolic alkalosis	↑	N	↑
Respiratory acidosis with renal compensation	↓ or N	↑	↑
Respiratory alkalosis with renal compensation	↑ or N	↓	↓
Metabolic acidosis with respiratory compensation	↓	↓	↓
Metabolic alkalosis with respiratory compensation	↑	↑	↑

Examining the chest

Examining the chest is a key skill for any clinician working in an environment where patients are unwell and may deteriorate.

An exam of the chest can tell us if there is:

- Constricted air flow.

- Fluid.

- Consolidation consistent with infective consolidation, atelectasis, fibrosis.

Consolidation is the space that normally contains air than now contains fluid or solid lung tissue.

Chest auscultation technique

Before you begin:

- Create as quiet an environment as possible.

- Patient sitting up with their chest not leaning on anything.

- Stethoscope should touch the patient's bare skin.

- Wet chest hair to decrease sounds caused by hair friction on the stethoscope.

When listening:

- Use the diaphragm of the stethoscope.

- Ask the patient not to speak.

- Ask the patient to breathe deeply through the mouth.

- Listen to one full breath in each location.

- Compare side to side.

Chest auscultation locations

There are 12 to 14 locations on the anterior and posterior respectively – listen to at least 6 locations.

Start at the apices, side to side to the bases. If there is a suspicious sound listen to nearby locations to assess the extent and character.

Locations are organised into categories based on intensity, pitch, location and inspiratory and expiratory ration.

Sounds are created by turbulent airflow. Expiratory breath sounds are quieter than inspiratory as the sound is going towards larger airways.

Chest auscultation locations

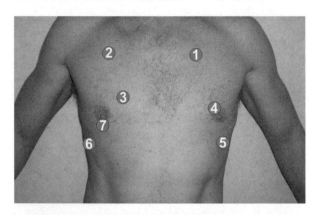

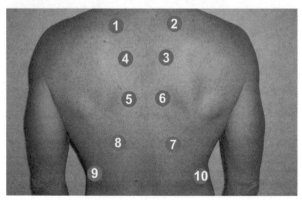

Normal sounds

Normal sounds: Tracheal and Bronchial

- Heard over trachea and main stem bronchi.

- Loud and high pitched.

- Heard over anterior chest wall second to fourth Intercostal Space (ICS) and third to sixth posterior.

Normal sounds: Other, also known as Vesicular

- Main normal breath sound is heard over most of the lungs.

- Soft and low pitched.

- Inspiratory sounds longer than expiratory sounds.

- May be softer in frail, elderly, obese or very muscular patients.

Normal sounds: Brochovesicular

- Best heard over the first and second ICS (Anterior Chest) and between the scapula (Posterior chest) – main stem bronchi.

- Pitch and duration is in between vesicular and bronchial.

Normal sounds: Bronchial

- Very loud and high pitched.

- Gap between inspiratory and expiratory phases of respiration.

- Expiratory sounds longer than inspiratory.

- Should only ever be heard over upper part of sternum, Manubrium like a handle, otherwise indicates consolidation.

Abnormal breath sounds

Bronchial breathing

- Bronchial breath sounds in abnormal locations.

- Louder than normal breath sounds.

- Heard when bronchi open into consolidated lung tissue, for example pneumonia.

Consolidation is the better transmission of sound than when the lungs are filled with air.

Diminished breath sounds

Breath sounds can be diminished even though they are not abnormal. They may be secondary to increased filtration of sounds such as pleural effusion or thickening.

Breath sounds can be diminished when there is decreased air movement. They will also be diminished when there is decreased movement of the chest.

Abnormal breath sounds: Diminished sounds

- Emphysema.

- Severe asthma.

- Pneumothorax.

- Atelectasis.

- Pleural Effusion.

- Acute Respiratory distress syndrome (ARDS) – later stages.

- Pain.

Causes of no breath sounds in an area of the chest include:

- Pleural effusion.

- Pneumothorax.

- Atelectasis, unless in the right upper lobe, adjacent tracheal sounds may be audible.

Adventitious sounds

- Are NOT changes to breath sounds.

- They are sounds that are added to normal breath sounds.

- Not heard over normal healthy lungs.

- Heard from lungs, pleura or pericardium.

- Can be discontinuous or continuous.

Discontinuous – Crackles

- Sound like – when hair is rubbed between fingers.

- Non musical brief sounds more commonly heard on inspiration.

Two explanations of mechanics:
Small airways open during inspiration and collapse during expiration causing crackle.
Air bubbles through secretions or partly closed airways during expiration.

Normal voice sounds

- Radiate through the airways and lungs out through the chest wall.

- Best heard over trachea and large airways but less well peripherally.

- Hard to understand individual words with stethoscope.

- With whispering, nothing is heard.

Abnormal voice sounds

Checking voice sounds can confirm or support diagnosis.

Bronchophony:

- Voice sounds increased and clearer but one cannot detect words.

- Heard under similar circumstances to bronchial breathing

Whispering pectoriloquy:

- Whispered words heard with a stethoscope.

- Heard under same circumstances as bronchial breath sounds and bronchophony.

Egophony:

- "E" is heard as "A" when listening through a stethoscope.

- Heard under same circumstances as bronchial breath sounds and bronchophony.

- Can also be heard if there is consolidation and pleural effusion.

Discontinuous crackles

- Timing described as early, mid or late inspiration or expiration.

- Pitch is described as high or low.

- Intensity as loud or soft.

- Also described as fine or coarse.

- Can disappear after a cough.

Adventitious sounds: Early and late inspiratory crackles

Late inspiratory crackles

- High pitched explosive sounds.

- Variable intensity.

- Most frequently heard over dependent or poorly ventilated lung regions.

Related conditions:

- Atelectasis (mucus plugging).

- Lobar pneumonia.

- Interstitial fibrosis.

- Pulmonary Oedema.

Early inspiratory crackles

Bronchitis

- Associated with excessive mucus production in patients with chronic bronchitis.

- Scanty and low pitched, not affected by position.

- Heard over all chest wall surfaces.

Bronchiectasis

- Irreversible dilatation of the bronchi in selected lung segments.

- Chronic & copious production of sputum.

- Fibrosis or atelectatic lung tissue surrounding the affected airway.

Causes

- Not heard over normal healthy lungs.

- Bacterial or viral pneumonia.

- Tumour.

- Foreign body obstruction.

- Tuberculosis.

- Chronic inflammatory or fibrotic lung disease.

Tend to be profuse crackles

Wheezes

Adventitious sounds: Continuous wheezes

- Produced when air flows through airways narrowed by secretions, foreign bodies or obstructive lesions.
- Continuous, high pitched sounds with a musical quality – Hissing
- Monophonic (one airway affected) or polyphonic (generalised obstruction).
- Inspiratory, expiratory or continuous.
- Longer duration than crackles.
- Can clear after a cough

Wheezes at the mouth, and breath sounds absent or diminished, signify impending respiratory failure.

Causes:

- Asthma.
- Chronic bronchitis.
- Chronic Obstructive Pulmonary Disease.
- Pulmonary Oedema.
- Congestive Cardiac Failure.
- Foreign body.
- Mucosal swelling.
- Tumour.

Stridor

- Loud musical monophonic wheeze.

- Can often be heard without stethoscope.

- Intensity distinguishes it from other monophonic wheezes.

- Usually inspiratory, however can be heard throughout respiratory cycle as airway constriction increases.

Stridor is a medical emergency – intubation or tracheotomy may be required

Causes:

- Severe upper respiratory infections.

- Laryngeal tumours.

- Tracheal stenosis.

- Whopping cough.

- Aspiration of foreign body.

If patient is drooling the epiglottis may be severely swollen. Do not examine the mouth as any stimulus may worsen the occlusion.

Pleural Rub

- When pleural surfaces are inflamed or roughened against each other.

- Creaking or brushing sound.

- Discontinuous or continuous.

- Can be localised to a particular place on the chest wall.

- Heard during inspiratory and expiratory phases.

Causes:

- Pleural effusion.

- Pneumothorax.

Chest auscultation key points

- Normal breath sounds, abnormal breath sounds and adventitious sounds.

- Assessing voice sounds may confirm thoughts of consolidation.

- Any crackles will alert you to a problem.

- Always find out the patient's medical condition.

- Use chest auscultation as an adjunct to overall diagnosis.

- Conditions are often not ideal for auscultation.

Ordering chest x-rays

The ordering of x-rays was once the prerogative of doctors alone. As the boundaries blur between the professions under the momentum of hospital at night project, nurse practitioners are embracing x-ray examination as an addition to their portfolio of skills.

If you are ordering x-rays as part of your role, ensure you are appropriately trained in the management of x-ray radiation. IR(ME)R is the recognised course.

Rationale for ordering a chest-xray:

- Confirmation of Central Venous Pressure (CVP) line placement.

- Confirmation of Naso-Gastric (NG) feeding tube placement.

- Necessary as an adjunct in diagnosis and treatment.

- Exclude respiratory pathology in patients with a shortness of breath.

Chest x-ray basic analysis

Patient's identity information
Date and time
Anterior Posterior (AP) or Posterior Anterior (PA) film
Technical quality

Check for rotation – was the patient correctly positioned when the x-ray was performed?

Technical assessment

- Assess the quality of x-ray penetration, you should just be able to see the lower thoracic vertebral bodies through the heart.

- Is the patient rotated? The spinous processes of the thoracic vertebrae should be midway between the medial ends of the clavicles.

- Most chest x-ray films are taken posterior anterior (PA) – that is, the x-rays shoot through from the back of the patient to the x-ray plate in front of the patient.

- PA films are better, particularly because the heart is not as magnified as on an AP film,

Chest x-ray abnormalities

- Consolidation related to infection or atelectasis.

- Lobe collapse.

- Pneumothorax.

- Pleural Effusion.

- Tumours and TB lesions.

- Pulmonary Oedema.

- Ventricular hypertrophy / cardiomegaly.

- Fractures.

- Widened mediastinum /aneurysm.

- Foreign objects.

- Air under the diaphragm

Other objects seen on a chest x-ray:

- CVP and other invasive lines.

- NG feeding tubes.

- Sternal wires.

- Prosthetic heart valves.

- Coronary artery stents.

- Pacemakers / Internal Cardiac Defibrillator.

- Tracheal tubes.

The normal chest x-ray with key anatomical features

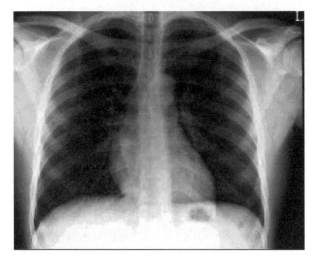

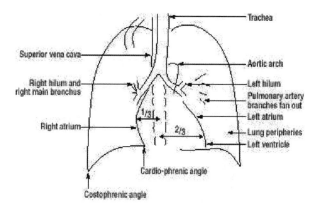

Trachea

Superior vena cava

Aortic arch

Right hilum and right main bronchus

Left hilum

Pulmonary artery branches fan out

1/3

2/3

Left atrium

Right atrium

Lung peripheries

Left ventricle

Cardio-phrenic angle

Costophrenic angle

The 10-point chest x-ray analysis approach

Point 1: Is there pathology of the bones?

Point 2: Is there evidence of pathology of the soft tissue of the chest wall?

Point 3: Is the trachea straight?

Point 4: Is the heart normal size? It should be less than half the width of the thorax. If the film is AP then it may appear larger.

Point 5: Is there mediastinal widening?

Point 6: Are the hila pull up or down? The left is higher than the right.

Point 7: Is the diaphragm raised? The right naturally sits higher than the left because it is above the liver.

Point 8: Are the lung fields free of shadowing?

Point 9: Are the costophrenic angles sharply defined?

Point 10: Is there good inspiration? The diaphragms should lie at the level of the sixth ribs anteriorly.

Closer look analysis

First look at the mediastinal contours – look down the left side and then up the right.

The trachea should be central.

The aortic arch is the first structure on the left, followed by the left pulmonary artery. The pulmonary artery branches fan out through the lung.

Two thirds of the heart lies on the left side of the chest, with one third on the right. The heart should take up no more than half of the thoracic cavity.

The left border of the heart is made up by the left atrium and left ventricle. The right border is made up by the right atrium alone. The right ventricle sits anteriorly and therefore does not have a border on the PA chest x-ray film.

Above the right heart border lies the edge of the superior vena cava.

The pulmonary arteries and main bronchi arise at the left and right hila. Enlarged lymph nodes can also occur here, as can primary tumours. These make the hilum seem bulky – the normal size of the hila on this film.

Now look at the lungs. Apart from the pulmonary vessels (arteries and veins), they should be black because of the radio translucence of air.

Look at both lungs, starting at the apices and working down, comparing left with right at the same level, just as you would when listening to the chest with your stethoscope.

Do not forget to look for a pneumothorax – in which case you would see the sharp line of the edge of the lung.

Make sure you can see the surface of the hemidiaphragms curving downwards and that the costophrenic and cardiophrenic angles are not blunted – suggesting an effusion.

Check there is no free air under the hemidiaphragm.

Chest x-ray examples – consolidation and tension pneumothorax

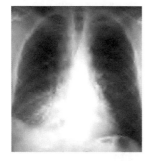

Consolidation is particularly evident in the diffuse opacity in the right base with blunting of costophrenic margin.

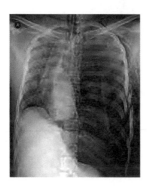

Tension pneumothorax

Chest x-ray Adenocarcinoma and pulmonary oedema

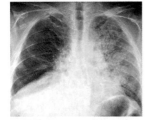

Adenocarcinoma

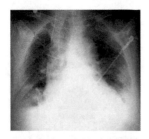

Pulmonary oedema example 1

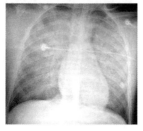

Pulmonary oedema example 2

Chest x-ray examples – Tumor, Right sided Pneumonia and Pleural Effusion

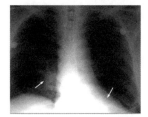

Tumor

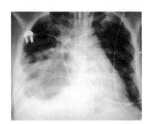

Right sided Pneumonia

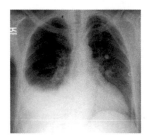

Pleural Effusion

Chapter 2 – Further reading

Chapter 2 – Further reading		
Barbara B	1995	A guide to physical examination and history taking. Sixth Edition, Lippincott, London.
Ruoss S and Schoene R Smith GB et al.	2005	The lung in extreme environments, an issue of clinics in chest medicine. Saunders, London.
Williams A J	1998	ABC of oxygen. Assessing and interpreting arterial blood gases and acid base balance. BMJ 1998:317:1212-6.
Gluck S L	1998	Acid-base. Electrolyte Quintet. The Lancet 1998:352:474-9.
Hess D	1986	Detection and monitoring of hypoxemia and oxygen therapy. Respiratory Care 2000:45:64-83.
Cooper, Nicola	2004	Acute Care: Arterial blood gases. BMJ 12:89-132.

Chapter 3

Advanced assessment – electrocardiogram interpretation

In this chapter the clinician will be guided in the taking of, and interpretation of, ECG recordings with a structure approach that allows the identification of abnormal or pathological rhythms.

In addition to, and as an adjunct to, the interpretation structure, examples are given that will enable the clinician to again to make a comparative analysis in practice.

Chapter 3 Contents

Chapter 3 Contents

ECG monitoring and rhythm strips

Cardiac monitors are available in most clinical areas within secondary care. They are easy to use and attach, and can alert the practitioner to life threatening arrhythmias and changes in a patient's cardiovascular status.

An ECG trace may be obtained with the electrodes attached in a variety of positions, ideally they are placed in a standard position each time so that abnormalities are easier to detect.

Monitors that have 3 leads are connected as follows:

Red – right arm or second intercostal space on the right of the sternum

Yellow – left arm or second intercostal space on the left of the sternum

Black or Green – left leg or more often in the region of the apex beat.

This will allow the Lead I, II or III configurations to be selected on the ECG monitor. Lead II is the most commonly used.

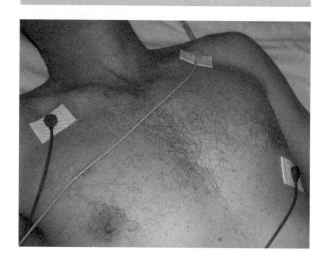

ECG and rhythm strip interpretation

It is useful to consider the ECG in terms of the activity of the heart as this will point the clinician in the direction of functional conception of the ECG recording.

The QRS complex has five distinct features with three waves that map to the function of the heart. The first is the "P" wave, which results from the movement of the depolarisation wave from the sino-atrial node. Atrial contraction follows the "P" wave some 0.1 seconds afterwards.

P = Atrial activity

The second wave of activity results from ventricular depolarisation and is quickly followed by ventricular contraction.

QRS = Ventricular activity

The third wave of activity is the repolarisation of the ventricles and this is seen as the "T" wave

T = Repolarisation of the ventricles

Normal ECG

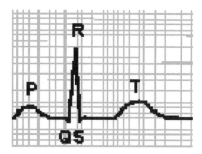

Five stage ECG monitor / Rhythm strip interpretation

1. Rate: What is the QRS rate?

2. Rhythm: Is the QRS rhythm regular or irregular?

3. Is the QRS width normal or prolonged?

4. Is there atrial activity present? If so what is it? Is there a normal "P" wave?

5. What is the relationship between atrial activity and ventricular activity?

RATE: To calculate the rate, divide 300 by the number of big squares per "R" to "R" interval

RHYTHM: If it is unclear whether the rate is regular or not, use a piece of card and mark three "R" waves and the move the card along and see if the marks match subsequent "R" waves.

Note: Complete irregularity = Atrial fibrillation (AF) or Ventricular fibrillation (VF)

Progressive irregularity = varying heart block

If AF is suspected remember there will be no discernable "P" waves and the QRS complexes are irregularly irregular.

However, atrial flutter has a saw tooth appearance.

Normal sinus rhythm

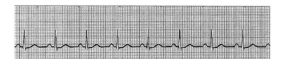

- Rate is 85 bpm.

- Rhythm is regular. Notice the distance between each "R" wave is the same.

- QRS duration is normal at less than 0.1 second, 2 1/2 small squares.

- "P" wave is visible before each QRS complex.

- P-R Interval is normal at less than 0.2 seconds, 5 small squares.

Sinus bradycardia

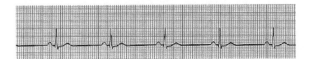

- Rhythm is regular.

- Rate is less than 60 beats per minute.

- QRS duration is normal.

- "P" wave is visible before each QRS complex.

- P-R interval is normal.

Sinus tachycardia

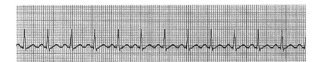

- Rate is more than 100 beats per minute.

- QRS duration is normal.

- "P" wave is visible before each QRS complex.

- P-R interval is normal.

Supraventricular tachycardia (Atrial tachycardia)

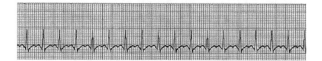

- Rate is between 140 and 220 beats per minute.

- Rhythm is regular.

- QRS duration is usually normal.

- "P" wave is often buried in preceding "T" wave.

- P-R Interval – depends on the site of supraventricular pacemaker

Atrial fibrillation (AF)

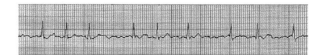

- Rate is usually between 100 and 160 beats per minute, but the rhythm is irregularly irregular.

- Slower rate if on medication.

- QRS duration is usually normal.

- "P" wave is not distinguishable as the atria are firing off all over.

- P-R interval is not measurable.

Atrial flutter

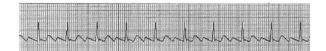

- Rate is around 110 beats per minute.

- Rhythm is regular.

- QRS duration is usually normal.

- "P" wave is replaced with multiple flutter waves ("F" waves), usually at a ratio of 2:1 (2 F to 1 QRS) but sometimes 3:1.

- "P" wave rate is 300 beats per minute.

- P-R interval is not measurable.

First degree AV block

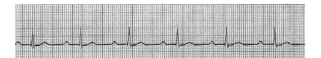

- Rate is normal.

- Rhythm is regular.

- QRS duration is normal.

- "P" wave – Ratio 1:1.

- "P" wave rate is normal.

- P-R Interval is prolonged (>5 small squares).

Second degree block type 1 (Wenckebach)

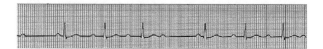

- Rate is normal or slow.

- Rhythm is regularly irregular.

- QRS duration is normal.

- "P" wave – Ratio 1:1 for 2, 3 or 4 cycles then 1:0.

- "P" wave rate is normal but faster than QRS rate.

- Progressive lengthening of P-R interval until a QRS complex is dropped.

Second degree block type 2)

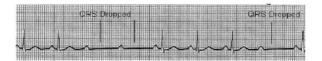

- Rate is normal or slow.

- Rhythm is regular.

- QRS duration is prolonged.

- "P" wave – Ratio 2:1 or 3:1.

- "P" wave rate is normal but faster than QRS rate.

- P-R Interval is normal or prolonged but constant.

Third degree block

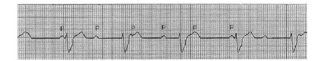

- Rate is slow.

- Rhythm is regular.

- QRS duration is prolonged.

- "P" wave is unrelated.

- "P" wave rate is normal but faster than the QRS rate.

- P-R interval – variation.

Bundle branch block

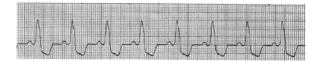

- Rate is normal.

- Rhythm is regular.

- QRS duration is prolonged.

- "P" wave – Ratio 1:1.

- P wave rate is normal and the same as QRS rate.

- P-R Interval – normal.

Premature ventricular complexes

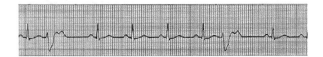

- Rate is normal.

- Rhythm is regular.

- QRS duration is normal.

- "P" wave – Ratio 1:1.

- "P" wave rate is normal and the same as the QRS rate.

- P-R interval is normal.

- You will also see 2 odd waveforms, these are the ventricles depolarising prematurely in response to a signal within the ventricles. Unifocal PVCs are shown above and multifocal PVCs are shown below.

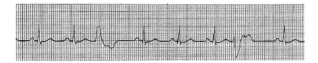

Junctional rhythms

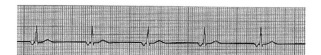

- Rate is between 40 and 60 beats per minute.

- Rhythm is regular.

- QRS duration is normal.

- "P" wave – Ratio 1:1, if visible and inverted in lead II.

- "P" wave rate is the same as the QRS rate.

- P-R interval is variable.

Below – Accelerated junctional rhythm

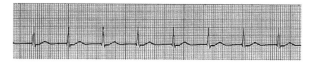

Ventricular Tachycardia (VT)

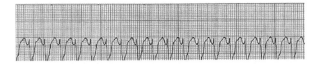

- Rate is between 180 and 190 beats per minute.

- Rhythm is regular.

- QRS duration is prolonged.

- "P" wave – Not seen.

Check pulse, if no pulse, will need defibrillation.

Ventricular Fibrillation (VF)

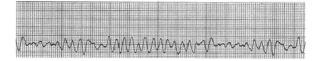

- Rate is more than 300 beats per minute and disorganised.

- Rhythm is irregular.

- QRS duration is not recognisable.

- "P" wave is not seen.

This patient needs to be defibrillated.

Asystole

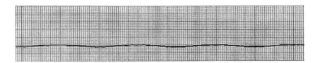

- Rate is 0 beats per minute.

- Rhythm is flat.

- QRS duration – None.

- "P" wave – None.

Check patient for breathing and pulse, check leads attached. **Carry out CPR**.

S-T Segment Elevation

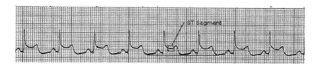

S-T segment elevation of above 2mm is not a normal finding on a monitor strip. You will see above that the S-T segment does not return to the base (isoelectric) line.

If this is seen on a monitor, a 12-lead ECG should be obtained to confirm diagnosis. The most common cause for this is acute myocardial infarction (see Chapter 8). However, Prinzmetal angina, or coronary artery spasm, and pericarditis are noted as other, but much less common, causes.

S-T Segment Depression

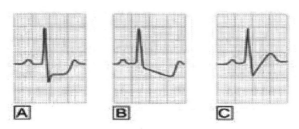

S-T segment depression can be observed in different forms. You will see above that the S-T segment is below the base line.

> A. Planar S-T depression – usually indicates myocardial ischcaemia.
>
> B. Down sloping depression also indicates ischcaemia.
>
> C. Up sloping depression may be a normal finding.

S-T depression is considered significant if the S-T segment is at least 1mm below the base line (measured 2mm beyond the QRS).

If this is seen on a monitor strip, a 12-lead ECG should be obtained to confirm diagnosis.

The shape of the S-T segment, and whether the abnormality is localised to leads looking at one area of the heart, often allows the cause of S-T depression to be diagnosed.

Although myocardial ischcaemia is a common cause of S-T depression, there are many other causes.

Causes of S-T Depression

- Tachycardia.

- Hypothermia.

- Hypokalemia.

- Bundle branch block.

- Non-Q wave (sub-endocardial) myocardial infarction.

- Reciprocal S-T elevation (showing an inverted view of what's happening at another place in the heart).

- Ventricular Hypertrophy.

- Digitalis (patient on long term or toxic from taking digoxin).

12-lead ECG and Acute Myocardial Infarction

An ECG is a graphical record of the activity of the heart. The 12-lead ECG is used extensively throughout healthcare. The main reason for recording all 12 leads is that it enhances pattern recognition.

The examination of a patient's ECG tracing, and analysing the rhythm, rate, conduction and contour patterns, allows the clinician to detect problems and facilitate an informed diagnosis.

Correct placement of the ECG electrodes

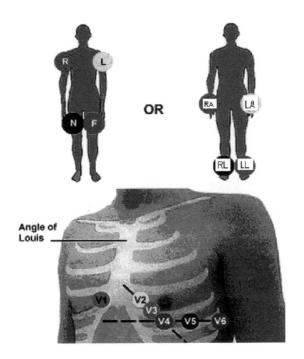

The logical way of the nurse interpreting a 12-lead ECG is to:

- Observe the rhythm strip first, normally lead II and at the bottom of the ECG, as described at the start of this chapter.

- Confirm the rate.

- Confirm the rhythm.

- Look for abnormalities in each territory of the heart such as "Q" waves, "T" wave inversion. Ignore lead AVR.

- Pay special attention to checking each territory for S-T segment elevation and S-T segment depression. If found in 2 leads in the same territory, acute myocardial infarction is likely.

The territories of the heart and the ECG leads that relate to them	
Anterior (Front)	I, V2 -V4
Septal	V1, V2
Inferior (Bottom)	II, III, AVF
Lateral (Left side)	AVL, V5, V6

Normal 12 lead ECG

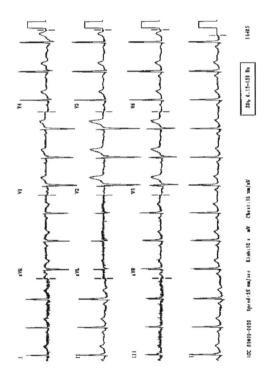

Acute Inferior Myocardial Infarction

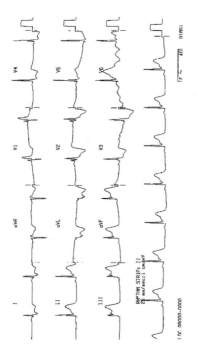

Notice the S-T segment elevation in leads II, III, and AVF, with reciprocal changes in AVL, V1-V4.

Acute Anterior Myocardial Infarction

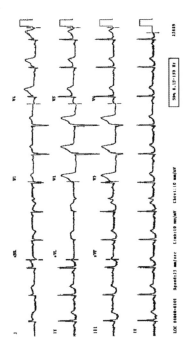

Notice the S-T segment elevation in leads I, V2, V3, V4, with reciprocal changes in III, AVF.

Acute Posterior Myocardial Infarction

In practice, posterior Myocardial Infarctions (back of the heart) are often misdiagnosed as unstable angina, as a standard 12-lead ECG does not have posterior leads.

In principle, S-T elevation is not commonly seen in this type of infarction. Key to diagnosis is the patient's history (particularly highlighting the symptoms of cardiac ischcaemia – see Chapter 8), and specific ECG changes of:

- Tall "R" wave in V1 – when the QRS is normally a negative deflection in this lead.

- Upright "T" waves especially in V2.

- S-T depression in V1 – V3.

Notice the positive "R" wave in V1 and S-T depression in V1-V3.

Chapter 3 – Further reading

Chapter 3: Further Reading		
Hampton J R	2003	The ECG made easy Toronto Churchill Livingston.
Houghton A R & Gray D	2003	Making sense of the ECG: a hands on guide Hodder headline group London.
Bennet D H	2002	Cardiac arrhythmias: Sixth Edition Arnold London.
Mackway-Jones K, Walker M	1999	A pocket guide for teaching medical instructors BMJ books, London.
Blomstrom-Lundqvist et al	2003	Guidelines for the management of the patient with supraventricular arrhythmias European heart journal24: 1857-1897.
International Liaison Committee on Resuscitation	2005	Acute coronary syndromes: emergency cardiovascular care science with treatment recommendations Resuscitation 2005:67:248-269.
Bertrand M E et al	2002	Management of acute coronary syndromes presenting without persistent ST segment elevation European heart journal 23:1809-1840.

Chapter 3: Further Reading

European society of cardiology Fox K A et al	2004	Management of acute myocardial infarction presenting with ST segment elevation European heart journal 24:28-66.
	2004	British cardiac working group on the definition of myocardial infarction Heart 90:603-609.
Mahoney B, Smith W	2005	Emergency interventions for hyperkalaemia Cochrane database system review CD 003235.

Chapter 4

The intravenous route

In the modern healthcare world the need to access the venous system is often paramount in the acute situation, and many therapeutic situations that are far from acute.

This chapter deals with accessing the venous system for the practitioner, in both instances of access for therapy or for venepuncture.

This chapter goes on to explore administration approaches and techniques, processes and systems for drug calculation and finally infection control as a key underpinning skill in the management of this invasive procedure.

Chapter 4 Contents

Cannulation

Cannulation is a key skill for any clinician whether in the emergency context of rapid vascular access being vital to the advanced resuscitation or as a prerequisite to the administration of key therapeutic intravenous agents.

As an advocate for the patient, the mastering of this specific area of expertise will protect the patient from the painful experience of multiple attempts at cannulation from inexpert and poorly skilled operatives.

This expertise, when truly mastered, is an enormous asset in propagating skills. Juniors, nursing and professions associated with medicine staff, as well trained staff, will more readily assimilate new taught skills and experience.

It is still not uncommon to hear of individuals being instructed in the "see one, do one, teach one" approach where the only clinical teaching deemed necessary to prepare for practice is one opportunity of observation.

Whilst the individual clinicians who have had this experience will often catch up through exposure to the task at hand and through contact with other colleagues, there will be an unnecessary period of poorly provisioned practice where patients will have a sub-optimal experience of cannulation.

When considering acquiring this skill and the likely deployment of this expertise, it is appropriate to consider those groups of patients who rely profoundly on the health and availability of their veins for what is often life saving care.

These groups are for example renal patients who rely on vascular access for haemodialysis treatment, oncology and haematology patients who need vascular access for a range of treatments and procedures and any patient who has a severe illness and needs advanced intervention.

In these patients the expertise of the practitioner in this area is vital.

Cannulation – Before the procedure

Before approaching the patient:

- Identify patient.

- Ensure rationale is still current. For example, should this patient still be taking IV antibiotics, or does this patient still require IV hydration.

- Gain informed consent.

Initial considerations before undertaking procedure:

- Patient's general circumstances – mental health or neuro-motor disorders, for example.

- Allergies to latex, plaster or tape.

- Fears and phobias.

- Faints.

- Clotting or bleeding disorders.

- Gather equipment.

- Wash hands.

- Apply tourniquet.

- Prepare and check equipment.

Cannulation – Equipment

- Gloves – the correct sizing is important.

- Tourniquet.

- Alcohol wipe or Chlorhexidine spray.

- Cotton wool or gauze and tape.

- Appropriate cannula dressing.

- Sharps bin.

- 5ml syringe.

- 5ml normal saline for flush.

- Choice of cannula:

    - Size 14 to 16g in Hypovolaemia.

    - Size 18g for blood, if possible.

    - Size 20 to 22g in all other cases.

The smaller the cannula gauge size, the wider the bore of the cannula.

Selection of the vein

- The selection of the vein is the most important part of the procedure.

- Make sure the patient and you are comfortable. Raise the bed or chair so you do not have to bend.

- Support the patient's arm on a pillow.

- Reassure the patient telling them that you will examine the arm first and warn them immediately before insertion of the cannula.

- Choose a site lower down the arm, unless the patient is likely to need aggressive fluids, is peri-arrest or in cardiac arrest, then the anti cubical fossa site is more appropriate.

- Palpate the vein to ensure it is elastic which is often described as bouncy.

- Note the path the vein takes.

- Note bends and changes in direction of the vein.

Cannulation – What to avoid

- Fibrosed veins which may appear to be a good place to site a cannula but on palpation are hard to the touch and inelastic.

- Inflamed veins

- Close to infection

- Bruising

- Directly over joints

- Side of CVA / post mastectomy

- Arm with infusion

- Dominant arm if possible

- Placing a cannula in the hand unless no other site is available. This position is very uncomfortable for the patient and extravasates easily due to the frequent movement of the patient's hand and of the cannula in the vein.

Cannulation – The procedure

- Apply tourniquet.

- Put on gloves.

- Clean and wait*

- Stretch skin with your thumb underneath the insertion site in order to stabilise the vein.

- Insert cannula, bevel up – 30 degrees. Use a slow and smooth action of when inserting.

- Obtain flashback. This is the movement of blood into the cannula port which tells you that you have breeched the vessel wall with the metal tip of the inner steel tube which runs down the middle of the cannula.

- The plastic catheter of the cannula itself is at this stage outside the vein as the steel protrudes beyond the catheter by a few millimetres.

- Stabilise cannula

- Advance the whole cannula a few millimetres.

- Advance the cannula catheter along the inner steel. The steel remains still whilst this happens.

- It is at this point that most failed cannulations occur as the inexperienced clinician will advance the catheter too early and it will buckle against the vessel wall.

The correct use of alcohol wipes is dependent on the clinician vigorously wiping the area for a minimum of one minute and then allowing at least one minute to dry.

In practice this often does not happen and the practice of "A quick wipe" can serve to agitate surface bacteria and in fact heighten the risk of infection being introduced at the time of cannulation.

Once in place

- Release tourniquet.

- Remove needle whist compressing the vein with your other hand.

- Dispose of sharps immediately.

- Attach a 3-way tap extension, flushed with normal saline, to cap-off.

- Secure with an appropriate dressing.

- Flush and confirm dressing.

- Dispose of contaminates.

- Document.

Cannulation – Difficulties

- Obese

- Dehydrated

- Elderly

- Very young

- Peripherally shut down

- Peripheral oedema

Cannulation – Hints and tips

- Ensure the tourniquet is applied tightly.

- Put tourniquet on before preparing equipment as it will allow greater time for the veins to fill.

- Tapping veins can help.

- Clenching and unclenching of the fist can make the veins more available.

- A hot compress using, for example, a small electric pad such as the type used for palliation of localised pain.

- A hot water dip can make the veins expand with the heat

Cannulation – Complications

- Infection localised to the insertion site.

- Systemic infection as septicaemia can be as a result of local infection.

- Extravasation is a common complication of intravenous therapy but in extreme cases, particularly where hypertonic solution is involved, can lead to tissue damage up to and including necrosis.

- Haematoma is also a common problem and usually occurs at the time of insertion. It is often related to poor technique of advancing the cannula catheter.

- Arterial puncture can occur if an unusual site is being explored in the difficult to cannulate patient. When this occurs strong and sustained pressure needs to be applied to the puncture site.

Venepuncture

Taking of blood is a skill that underpins advanced assessment and should be considered an adjunct to the advanced and enhanced level practice.

The taking of blood should not be considered a stand alone task where the practitioner has no investment or indeed rationale with regard to the results of the ordered blood tests.

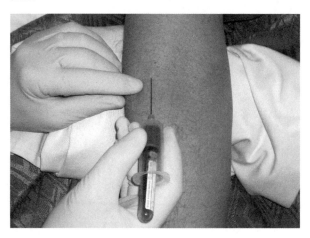

Venepuncture – The procedure

- Apply tourniquet.

- Put on gloves.

- Have the correct, and correctly labelled, bottles.

- Clean and wait*

- Stretch the skin with your thumb underneath the insertion site in order to stabilise the vein.

- Insert butterfly or needle, bevel up – 30 degrees using a slow and smooth action of insertion.

- Obtain flashback. The butterfly has an advantage over fixed needle systems as the difficult and small vein can be more readily found with a butterfly and there is no vacuum to collapse the vein in this system.

Refer to the cannulation section for more information regarding vein selection and location.

Venepuncture with the vacutainer system

The vacutainer system has been designed to reduce the risk of an infected needlestick injury, by having enclosed sharp filling system with blood bottles pre-charged with vacuum.

When this system is used correctly, the only exposed sharp is that which is inserted into the vein which is immediately disposed of into specifically designed sharps bins.

A problem can occur when this system is not used correctly, or when not all elements are available, and the practitioner chooses to fill the vacuum charged bottles with a syringe and needle which has been used to take the blood.

This practice is dangerous as the practitioner is pointing a potentially infected needle towards their own hand, which increases the risk of a dirty needlestick injury considerably.

Blood Bottles

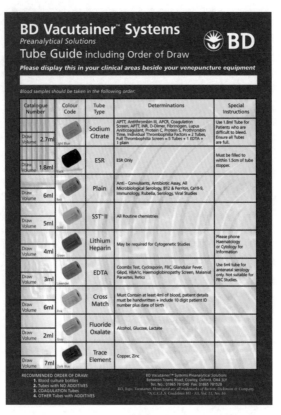

BD Vacutainer™ Systems
Preanalytical Solutions

BD

Tube Guide including Order of Draw

Please display this in your clinical areas beside your venepuncture equipment

Blood samples should be taken in the following order:

Catalogue Number	Colour Code	Tube Type	Determinations	Special Instructions
Draw Volume 2.7ml	Light Blue	Sodium Citrate	APTT, Antithrombin III, APCR, Coagulation Screen, APTT, INR, D-Dimer, Fibrinogen, Lupus Anticoagulant, Protein C, Protein S, Prothrombin Time, Individual Thrombophilia Factors = 2 Tubes, Full Thrombophilia Screen = 5 Tubes + 1 EDTA + 1 plain	Use 1.8ml Tube for Patients who are difficult to bleed. Ensure all Tubes are full.
Draw Volume 1.8ml	Black	ESR	ESR Only	Must be filled to within 1.5cm of tube stopper.
Draw Volume 6ml	Red	Plain	Anti - Convulsants, Antibiotic Assay, All Microbiological Serology, B12 & Ferritin, Ca19-9, Immunology, Rubella, Serology, Viral Studies	
Draw Volume 5ml	Gold	SST™ II	All Routine chemistries	
Draw Volume 4ml	Green	Lithium Heparin	May be required for Cytogenetic Studies	Please phone Haematology or Cytology for Information
Draw Volume 3ml	Lavender	EDTA	Coombs Test, Cyclosporin, FBC, Glandular Fever, G6pd, HbA1c, Haemoglobinopathy Screen, Malarial Parasites, Retics	Use 6ml tube for antenatal serology only. Not suitable for FBC Studies.
Draw Volume 6ml	Pink	Cross Match	Must Contain at least 4ml of blood, patient details must be handwritten + include 10 digit patient ID number plus date of birth	
Draw Volume 2ml	Grey	Fluoride Oxalate	Alcohol, Glucose, Lactate	
Draw Volume 7ml	Dark Blue	Trace Element	Copper, Zinc	

RECOMMENDED ORDER OF DRAW:
1. Blood culture bottles
2. Tubes with NO ADDITIVES
3. COAGULATION Tubes
4. OTHER Tubes with ADDITIVES

BD Vacutainer™ Systems Preanalytical Solutions
Between Towns Road, Cowley, Oxford. OX4 3LY
Tel. No.: 01865 781540 Fax: 01865 781528
BD, logo, Vacutainer, Hemogard are all trademarks of Becton, Dickinson & Company.
N.C.C.L.S. Guidelines H1 - A3, Vol. 11, No. 16.

Needlestick injury

A needlestick injury is any injury where the skin has been breeched with an infected sharp. This can include grazes as well as puncture wounds.

Similarly, splashes of blood or blood stained fluid into the eye is considered as carrying the same risk but of a different order.

Following a mucocutaneous exposure, via the mucous membrane, the average risk is estimated to be less than one in one thousand.

Where intact skin is exposed to HIV infected blood, no risk of HIV transmission is considered.

A needlestick injury is an emergency.

- Stop what you are doing immediately.

- Force the wound to bleed.

- Wash under running water.

- Report immediately to your immediate manager.

- Go directly to Accident and Emergency.

Report your injury to the triage nurse who will award an urgent category.

Needlestick injury and Post Exposure Prophylaxis (PEP)

Consider with the Accident and Emergency clinician whether or not to take PEP.

This is a short course, generally around three months, of anti-retroviral triple therapy which is thought to be of value in preventing seroconversion when an individual has been exposed to the HIV infection.

The most usual regime offered is a three drug combination of:

- AZT

- 3TC

- Indinavir or Nelfinavir

These drugs are started immediately.

A case control study amongst healthcare workers exposed to HIV has found that the administration of AZT for four weeks after exposure was associated with an 80% reduced risk of seroconversion.

AZT treatment at this stage is believed to block the infection of immune system cells by HIV, so prompt AZT treatment is likely to block the establishment of HIV infection in an individual who has been exposed to the virus.

It is assumed that a combination of two or three drugs may be even more effective than AZT alone at blocking HIV infection.

The decision to commence PEP

Risk assessment:

- Was the donor patient HIV positive?

- Was the patient known have a high viral load at the time of inoculation?

- Was the injury received a deep injury from large diameter needle?

It must be remembered that despite the benefits of PEP, there is evidence that the standard regimen of AZT, 3TC and Indinavir is poorly tolerated.

Nine out of 18 healthcare workers at three London hospitals who commenced this regimen stopped or changed therapy due to side effects within four weeks.

Six of the nine who started Indinavir required more than two weeks off work. Among the other 9, only one required more than 7 days' leave. There were no discontinuations among the five people who received saquinavir (Parkin).

PEP – Department of Health guidance

If exposed in the course of your work you may well have access to triple therapy on site which could save time.

Local policy will include instructions to inform occupational health in the instance of exposure.

Training on prevention of needlestick injuries and post exposure procedures, including AZT treatment, should also be included.

Speed of administration of PEP: It is assumed that PEP needs to be administered within 24 hours of exposure, and

July 2000: NHS Trusts, or other healthcare settings, should develop a post-exposure policy.

Starter packs of triple therapy should be available on site for use following occupational exposure.

is most likely to be most efficacious if started within one hour of exposure.

Drug administration

The pharmaceutical management of a patient infers two distinct responsibilities and functions which fall to different professions at different times. These are prescribing the right drug and giving the right drug correctly.

Nurses are now in the position of fulfilling both of these roles and many nurses have encountered drugs as the clinician who dispenses them, secondary to the prescription of a medical colleague. However, this is now changing with the nurse also prescribing, which will become much more the case following the changes to nurse prescribing that came into effect in April 2006.

Whatever role the nurse fills, there are many common elements to both functions, namely giving the correct drug to the correct patient for the correct reason.

Whether dispensing or prescribing a drug, it is absolutely essential that all the team involved are able to competently calculate and give the correct dose.

What follows is guidance on good practice for prescribing and dispensing, a break down of the units of measurement and an approach to drug calculations.

When giving drugs remember the following check list:

- Name

- Date

- Time

- Route

- Allergies

- Interactions with other prescribed drugs

- Correct dose

- Appropriate drug for this patient with this condition

Système International (SI)

Système International Units		
Mass		
1 kilogram (kg)	=	1,000 grams
1 gram (g)	=	1,000 milligrams
1 milligram (mg)	=	1,000 micrograms
1 microgram (μg)	=	1,000 nanograms (ng)
Volume		
1 litre	=	1,000 millilitres (ml)
1 millilitre	=	1,000 microlitres (μg)

Abbreviations **must not** be used in the writing of prescriptions as there is a high possibility of confusion with other abbreviations.

Making a calculation – First method

This method enables the nurse to give the correct dose by identifying the strength of the solution per volume. From this point a calculation is done to identify the specific volume needed for the prescribed dose.

Example 1

A dose of 100mgs has been prescribed. However, the drug is only available in strengths and volume of 400mg in 5ml.

Step 1

Calculate the dose per ml:

$$\frac{400 \text{ mg}}{5 \text{ ml}} = 80 \text{ mg/ml}$$

This preparation therefore has a strength of 80mg per ml.

To achieve a dose of 100mg we have to do the following calculation

$$\frac{100 \text{ mg} \times 1\text{ml}}{80 \text{ mg/ml}} = 1.25\text{ml}$$

First method continued

This calculation shows that 80 goes into 100 once and leave a remainder of 20.

80 doesn't go into 20 but does go into 200, 2.5 times.

```
      1 r 20
  _____
80/100
```

```
     2. 5
  _____
80/200
```

The answer therefore is 1 + 2.5 = 1.25mls of solution.

Making a calculation – Second method

This second approach is based on a concept of relationships between proportions.

> The formula
>
> Dose required (mg)
>
> ——————————————— X   Dose volume (ml) of
>
> Strength available (mg)   available product
>
> = Volume (ml) containing the required dose

Therefore, as with the previous example:

Dose required = 100 mgs
——————————————————
         x 5mls

Strength available 400mg

= 100 divided by 400 = 0.25 x 5 = 1.25mls

Second method continued

> This formula can more easily be described
>
>   X   volume available
>
> What you've got

Chapter 4 – Further reading

Chapter 4: Further Reading		
Dougherty L & Lister S	2005	The Royal Marsden Hospital Manual of Clinical Nursing Procedures – Sixth edition Blackwell, London.
Audit Commission	2001	A spoonful of sugar: Medicines management in the NHS hospitals, Audit Commission, London.
BMA & RPS	2003	British National Formulary British Medical Association & Roya Pharmaceutical Association, London.
Barbara B	1995	A Guide to Physical Examination and History Taking, Sixth Edition, Lippincott, London.
Creswell J	1999	1999 Nurse prescribing handbook Association of nurse prescribing and community nurse UK.
DOH	1999	Review of prescribing, supply and administration of medicines: Final report Crown three, The Stationary Office, London.
Hyde L	2002	Legal and professional aspects of intravenous therapy. Nursing Standard 15(26), 39-42

Chapter 4: Further Reading

Lonsway R	2001	IV therapy in the home, Infusion therapy in clinical practice WB Saunders, Philadelphia.
Weinstein S M	2000	Plummer's principles and practices of intravenous therapy. Seventh edition Lippincott, Philadelphia.

Chapter 5

Blood test interpretation and values

This chapter details the expected values for a number of the more common blood tests, with brief interpretations of what a high or low value could mean to the bedside clinician.

The purpose of the explanations is to point the practitioner in the right direction with regard to an impression that the first glance may give. Where blood tests have an integral relationship with therapy and management, this information has also been included.

This chapter is further intended to enable the clinician as an aid, or as a pointer in the right direction, for interpretation and subsequent management planning. It is not intended to give a complete or comprehensive interpretation of the significance of the blood test result.

The format of this chapter follows a structure where blood tests are grouped according to body system or function and they are presented as a highlighted section within the greater range of common blood tests. This is to accommodate bedside interpretation where reference to many tests may be needed concurrently.

Embedded within the text, there is also a guide to the likely bottles used for each test. It must be remembered that this can vary and should be compared to local guidelines from your place of work.

Chapter 5 Contents

Simple Haematology blood test results

Haemoglobin Hb	Men 13 - 18 g/dl W 11.5 - 16 g/dl
Mean cell volume MCV	76 - 96 fl
White cells (Total)	WCC 4 - 11 x 10 ^{9}/L
Neutrophils	2 - 7.5 x 10 ^{9}/L
Lymphocytes	1.3 - 3.5 x 10 ^{9}/L
Eosinophils	0.04 - 0.44 x 10 ^{9}/L

Urea and electrolytes

Sodium	135 - 145 mmol/L
Potassium	3.5 - 5.0 mmol/L
Creatinine	70 - 150 µmol/L
Urea	2.5 - 6.7 mmol/L
Calcium	2.12 - 2.65 mmol/L
Albumin	35 - 50 g/L
Proteins	60 - 80 g/L

Liver function tests

Bilirubin	3 - 17 µmol/L
Alanine aminotransferase (ALT)	3 - 35 iu/L
Aspartate transaminase (AST)	3 - 35 iu/L
Alkaline phosphatase	30 - 300 iu/L

Simple Haematology blood test results

Blood Test	Range	Implications
Haemoglobin **Hb** **Purple Bottle** 	Men 13-8g/dl	**Low** Anaemia Blood loss Haemodilution
	W 11.5-16gdl	**High** Polycythaemia Dehydration

Blood Test	Range	Implications
White cell count **WCC Purple bottle**	4 -11x 10(9)/L	

Simple Haematology blood test results

Blood Test	Range	Implications
Neutrophils **Purple Bottle**	2 - 7.5 x 10(9)	**Low** • Viral infections • Hyperspleenism • SLE • Rheumatoid arthritis • B12 deficiency • Folate deficiency • Sulfonamides • Carbimazole **High** • Viral infections • Inflammation • Infarction • Burns • Bleeding • Trauma • Widespread malignancy • Leukaemias

Simple Haematology blood test results

Blood Test	Range	Implications
Lymphocytes **Purple Bottle**	1.3 - 3.5 x 10(9)/L	**Low** • SLE • Uraemia • AIDs • Following chemotherapy • Following radiotherapy • Steroid therapy **High** • Viral infections • Toxoplasmosis • Whooping cough • Chronic lymphatic Leukaemias

Simple Haematology blood test results

Blood Test	Range	Implications
Eosinophils **Purple Bottle** 	0.04 - 0.44 x 10(9)/L	**High** • Asthma • Skin diseases (Uticarias) • Leukaemias • Adrenal insufficiency • Following infection • End organ damage

Simple haematology blood test results

Blood Test	Range	Implications
Monocytes **Purple Bottle** 	0.2 - 0.8 x 10(9)/L	**High** • Acute and ahronic infections • Malignancy • Acute myeloid leukaemia • Hodgkin's disease

Blood Test	Range	Implications
Basophils **Purple Bottle** 	0.0 - 0.1 x 10(9)/L	**High** • Viral infections • Malignancy • Uticarias • Myxoedema • Post spleenectomy

Simple haematology blood test results

Blood Test	Range	Implications
Mean cell volume (MCV) 1.3 - 3.5 x 10(9)/L **Purple Bottle** 	76 - 96fl	**High** • Drugs • Alcohol, azathioprine, • Zidovudine • Haemolysis • Liver disease • Hypothyroidism • Myeodyssplasia • Macrocytic anaemia • MCV> 110 • Vitamin B12 deficiency • Hydoxycarbamide

Simple haematology blood test results

Blood Test	Range	Implications
Platelets	150 -400x10(9)/L	**Low – known as thrombo cytopenia** • Aplastic anaemia's • Bone marrow infiltration • Pancytopenia • Platelets below 40 the patient is at great risk of bleeding **High** • Commonly related to infection

Urea and electrolytes blood test results

Blood Test	Range	Implications
Sodium (Na)	135 - 145 mmol/L	**Low** Sodium loss with low urine sodium • Addison disease • Diuretic stage of renal failure • Osmolar diuresis ↑glucose or ↑urea • Diarrhoea • Fistula Sodium loss with high urine sodium • Nephritic syndrome • Cirrhosis • Renal failure **High** Fluid loss without replacement • Dehydration • Diarrhoea • Vomiting burns High sodium content in infusion • Diabetes incipidus • Osmotic diuresis • Aldosteronism

Blood Test	Range	Implications
Potassium K+ *An erroneously high K+ can be seen in a blood sample which has haemolysed, due to red cell trauma leaking intracellular potassium in to serum.*	3.5 - 5.0 mmol/L	**Low** • Diuretics • D&V • Pyloric stenosis • GI fistulae • Cushing's • Alkalosis • Renal tubular failure **High** • Oliguric renal failure • Excessive K+ therapy • Rhabdomyolysis • Metabolic acidosis (DM) • Addison's disease • Large amount blood transfusion • K+ sparing diuretics • ACE inhibitors • Suxamethonium

Potassium lower than 2.5 **needs urgent intervention** and is a life threatening.

Potassium greater than 6.5 **needs urgent intervention** and is a life threatening.

Urea and electrolytes blood test results

Blood Test	Range	Implications
Urea	2.5- 6.7 mmol/L	**Low** • Low protein diet • Immediately post haemodialysis **High** • Renal insufficiency • Haemo concentration in severe dehydration

Urea and electrolytes blood test result

Blood Test	Range	Implications
Calcium	2.12 - 2.65 mmol/L	**Low Calcium** Hypocalcaemia • Tetany • Neuro excitability **High** • High serum calcium can correlate to bone disease

Urea and electrolytes blood test results

Blood Test	Range	Implications
Albumin *Low albumin causes oedema*	35 - 50 g/L	**Low** • Nephrotic syndrome • Liver disease • Malabsorption • Malnutrition **High** • Dehydration artefact

Blood Test	Range	Implications
Proteins 	60 - 80 g/L	**Low** • As albumin **High** • As albuminct

Liver function tests

Blood Test	Range	Implications
Bilirubin	3 - 17 µmol/L	**High** Jaundice Viable at a level > 35µmol/L

Blood Test	Range	Implications
Alanine aminotransferase **ALT**	3-35iu/L	**High** Indicates hepatocyte damage: Disease of the liver causing jaundice

Blood Test	Range	Implications
Aspartate transaminase **ALT**	3-35iu/L	**High** Indicates hepatocyte damage: Disease of the liver causing jaundice

Liver function tests

Blood Test	Range	Implications
Alkaline phosphatase	30-300 iu/L	**High** May indicate obstructive jaundice but found with other conditions such as malignant infiltration

Cardiac enzymes

There are a collection of enzymes and proteins that, when measured, can give useful information on the likelihood of a patient having suffered a myocardial infarction (See Chapter 3).

This is of interest since the emergence of Thrombolysis therapy where diagnosis cannot be made on ECG alone (See Chapter 3).

There has been further pressure on the development of a reliable test which will enable a definitive statement that the patient has not suffered from a myocardial infarction and can be safely discharged home. This is the pressure to be ever more efficient in the use hospital beds.

Troponin T, or more commonly Trop T, is currently the test of choice for many acute hospital environments.

Troponin T

Troponin T rises between 4 and 8 hours in most patients. However, some patients will not show a rise until up to 12 hours.

Tests for Troponin T are insensitive within 6 hours of symptoms.

A negative Troponin T result can effectively rule out myocardial infarction if drawn at or more than 12 hours after symptom onset.

Troponin T will normally remain raised for between 7 and 14 days.

Cardiac enzymes	
CK	Creatine kinase
CK-MB	CK Cardiac Isoenzyme
AST	Aspartate transaminase
LDH	Lactate dehydrogenase

CK is found in myocardial muscle and skeletal muscle, and can be elevated from non-myocardial source. If you are in any doubt measure CK MB.

CK MB is more specific marker for myocardial infarction and will rise up to 12 hours or so post injury and fall away to dissipation by day 3. It is therefore a useful marker for new or subsequent injury.

Enzyme levels and peaks	
CK can rise to 5 times the normal level	Peaks at day 3
CK-MB rises to 4 times normal level	Peaks at day 2
AST rises to 3 times normal level	Peaks at day 3
LDH rises to 3 times normal level	Peaks at day 3

Anti coagulation and treatment protocol

Indication for therapy:

- DVT.

- Pulmonary emboli.

- Arterial fibrillation (See Chapters 3 and 5).

- Cerebral vascular accident (CVA) prevention.

- Prophylactic pre and post operatively, maybe given in prolonged bed rest.

Low molecular weight heparin is more predictable in its effect than standard heparin so can be given twice daily without need of monitoring.

Prophylaxis of DVT prior to surgery:

- Dalteparin sodium.

- 2,500 units subcutaneous 1 to 2 hours before surgery.

- 2,500 units once daily for 5 to 7 days.

High risk prophylaxis of DVT prior to surgery 1:

- Dalteparin sodium.

- 2,500 units subcutaneous 1 to 2 hours before surgery.

- 2,500 units 8 to 12 hours later.

High risk prophylaxis of DVT prior to surgery 2:

- Dalteparin sodium.

- 5,000 units subcutaneous the evening before surgery.

- 5,000 units once daily for 5 to 7 days.

Treatment of DVT and Pulmonary Emboli with subcutaneous Dalteparin sodium low molecular weight heparin.

Weight	Dose
46 to 56kg	10,000 units
57 to 68kg	12,500 units
69 to 82kg	15,000 units
83kg and above	18,000 units

Standard or unfractionated heparin

Treatment for DVT:

- Initial dose IV 5,000iu

- Continuous infusion of 15 to 25 iu per kg per hour

- Or subcutaneous heparin 15,000 iu twice daily

Assembly:

- 25,000 iu heparin to gross volume 50ml with normal saline 0.9%

- Strength 500 iu per ml

Infused at between 2 and 4ml per hour, titrated to activated partial prothrombin time (APTT). Monitoring APTT every 10 hours.

APTT	Change rate by units per hour
5 to 7	-500
4 to 5	-300
3 to 4	-100
2.5 to 3	-50
1.5 to 2.5	0
1.2 to 1.4	+200
Less than 1.2	+400

If APTT is greater than 7, stop IV and check again in 4 hours.

Chapter 5 – Further reading

Chapter 5: Further Reading

Barbara B,	1995	A Guide to physical examination and history taking. Sixth Edition Lippincott, London.
Dougherty L & Lister S	2005	The Royal Marsden Hospital Manual of Clinical Nursing Procedures Sixth Edition Blackwell, London.
Fletcher J& Batiste P	1997	Incidence of deep vein thrombosis following vascular surgery International Angioology 16(1): 65-68.
Huw Llewelyn, et al	2006	Oxford Handbook of Clinical Diagnosis Oxford Handbooks S.
Michael McGee	2003	A Guide to Laboratory Investigations Radcliffe Medical Press

Chapter 6

The 2005 adult resuscitation guidelines

The new guidelines for resuscitation were published on the 27 November 2005, with a plan to implement these new guidelines over time. This is due to some of the significant changes involved in the reconfiguration of machinery that is dependant on the resources outside of the direct control of many healthcare providers.

It is planned for the distribution of adult related education materials to be in place by April 2006 with paediatric and neonatal following this. It is reasonable to assume that many healthcare providers will use April 2006 as the start date for the use of the new guidelines. However many Trusts, PCTs and other progressive environments may begin before this time.

It has been recognised by the Resuscitation Council (UK) that the implementation of the new guidelines will happen over time and inevitably there will be a period of overlap in which case clinicians in practice should ensure a consensus at the bedside.

This chapter is a faithful reproduction of the new guidelines in algorithm format as a quick reference guide for the busy clinician.

Chapter 6 Contents

The adult basic life support algorithm

Resuscitation Council (UK) 2005

Adult Basic Life Support

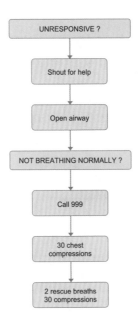

Treatment for adult choking

Resuscitation Council (UK) 2005

Adult choking treatment

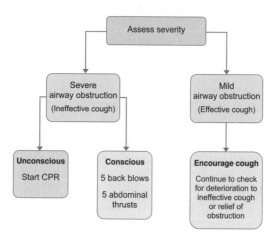

In-hospital resuscitation

Resuscitation Council (UK) 2005

In-hospital resuscitation

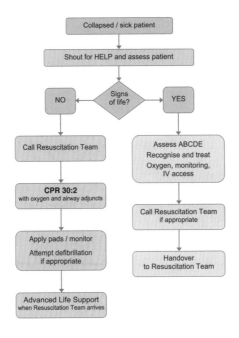

AED algorithm

Resuscitation Council (UK) 2005

AED Algorithm

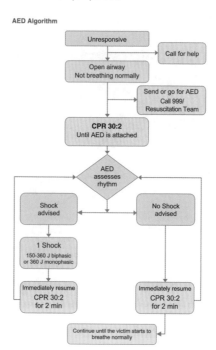

174

Adult advanced life support algorithm

Resuscitation Council (UK) 2005

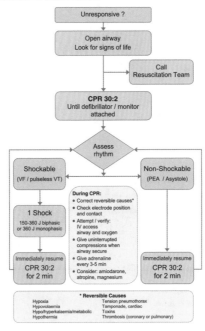

Adult Advanced Life Support Algorithm

Unresponsive ?

Open airway
Look for signs of life

Call
Resuscitation Team

CPR 30:2
Until defibrillator / monitor
attached

Assess
rhythm

Shockable
(VF / pulseless VT)

Non-Shockable
(PEA / Asystole)

During CPR:
- Correct reversible causes*
- Check electrode position and contact
- Attempt / verify:
  IV access
  airway and oxygen
- Give uninterrupted compressions when airway secure
- Give adrenaline every 3-5 min
- Consider: amiodarone, atropine, magnesium

1 Shock

150-360 J biphasic
or 360 J monophasic

Immediately resume

CPR 30:2
for 2 min

Immediately resume

CPR 30:2
for 2 min

* Reversible Causes	
Hypoxia	Tension pneumothorax
Hypovolaemia	Tamponade, cardiac
Hypo/hyperkalaemia/metabolic	Toxins
Hypothermia	Thrombosis (coronary or pulmonary)

Bradycardia algorithm

Resuscitation Council (UK) 2005

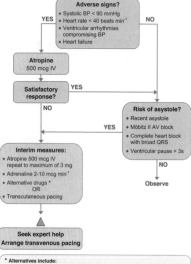

Bradycardia Algorithm
(includes rates inappropriately slow for haemodynamic state)

If appropriate, give oxygen, cannulate a vein, and record a 12-lead ECG

Adverse signs?
- Systolic BP < 90 mmHg
- Heart rate < 40 beats min⁻¹
- Ventricular arrhythmias compromising BP
- Heart failure

YES / NO

Atropine
500 mcg IV

Satisfactory response? — YES

NO

Risk of asystole?
- Recent asystole
- Möbitz II AV block
- Complete heart block with broad QRS
- Ventricular pause > 3s

YES / NO

Interim measures:
- Atropine 500 mcg IV repeat to maximum of 3 mg
- Adrenaline 2-10 mcg min⁻¹
- Alternative drugs *
  OR
- Transcutaneous pacing

Observe

Seek expert help
Arrange transvenous pacing

*Alternatives include:
    Aminophylline
    Isoprenaline
    Dopamine
    Glucagon (if beta-blocker or calcium-channel blocker overdose)
    Glycopyrrolate can be used instead of atropine

Tachycardia algorithm

Resuscitation Council (UK) 2005

Tachycardia Algorithm (with pulse)

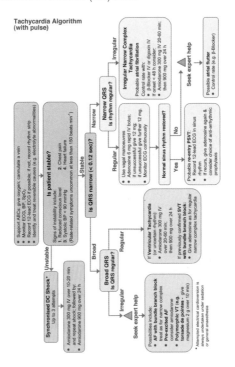

* Support ABCs: give oxygen; cannulate a vein
* Monitor ECG, BP, SpO₂
* Record 12-lead ECG if possible; if not, record rhythm strip
* Identify and treat reversible causes (e.g. electrolyte abnormalities)

Is patient stable?

Signs of instability include:
1. Reduced conscious level
2. Chest pain
3. Systolic BP < 90 mmHg
4. Heart failure

(Rate-related symptoms uncommon at less than 150 beats min⁻¹)

Unstable

Synchronised DC Shock*
Up to 3 attempts

* Amiodarone 300 mg IV over 10–20 min and repeat shock; followed by:
* Amiodarone 900 mg over 24 h

Stable

Is QRS narrow (< 0.12 sec)?

Broad → **Broad QRS Is QRS regular?**

Irregular → Seek expert help

Possibilities include:
* AF with bundle branch block treat as for narrow complex
* Pre-excited AF consider amiodarone
* Polymorphic VT (e.g. torsade de pointes – give magnesium 2 g over 10 min)

Regular

If Ventricular Tachycardia (or uncertain rhythm):
* Amiodarone 300 mg IV over 20–60 min;
* then 900 mg over 24 h

If previously confirmed SVT with bundle branch block:
* Give adenosine as for regular narrow complex tachycardia

Narrow → **Narrow QRS Is rhythm regular?**

Regular

* Use vagal manoeuvres
* Adenosine 6 mg rapid IV bolus; if unsuccessful give 12 mg; if unsuccessful give further 12 mg.
* Monitor ECG continuously

Normal sinus rhythm restored?

Yes → Probable re-entry PSVT:
* Record 12-lead ECG in sinus rhythm
* If it recurs, give adenosine again & consider choice of anti-arrhythmic prophylaxis

No

Seek expert help

Possible atrial flutter
* Control rate (e.g. β-Blocker)

Irregular → **Irregular Narrow Complex Tachycardia**
Probable atrial fibrillation

Control rate with:
* β-Blocker IV or digoxin IV
If onset < 48 h consider:
* Amiodarone 300 mg IV 20–60 min; then 900 mg over 24 h

* Attempted electrical cardioversion is always undertaken under sedation or general anaesthesia

Summary of key changes within the 2005 adult guidelines

- Assessment of breathing: *Not breathing normally and not responding* rather than the previous assessment finding of *No breathing*.

- Chest compressions begin before rescue breaths.

- The rate and ratio of chest compressions has changes to 30:2.

- Place hands at the centre of the chest rather than the more complex previous method.

- Giving each rescue breath over 1 second only.

- Single shock strategy to defibrillation.

Rationale for key changes within the 2005 adult guidelines

Assessment of breathing

The designation not breathing normally has replaced the term and finding of not breathing. It was identified by the Resuscitation Council (UK) that agonal breathing had not been previously identified and commencement of resuscitation was often delayed.

Chest compressions begin before rescue breaths

The rationale for this change reflected two new insights. The first insight is that in an arrest not preceded by hypoxia, there is a degree of residue oxygenated blood. If circulated, this blood is of value in terms of resuscitation with chest compressions alone, or with chest compressions as a priority.

The second insight is that resuscitation was often delayed as rescuers were reluctant to do mouth to mouth and consequently do nothing.

With the layperson that is reluctant to do mouth to mouth, then chest compression only resuscitation is advised with a rate of 100 compressions per minute.

The rate and ratio of chest compressions has changed to 30:2

The rational for this change is related to the known correlation between poor outcome and interruption in chest compressions and it was felt this change brought the BLS algorithm closer to the ideal of continuous uninterrupted chest compressions.

Hand placement

The placement of hands when giving chest compressions has also changed to the placement being at the centre of the chest rather than the more time consuming and more complex previous method.

Rescue breaths

The time spent giving rescue breaths has also change to giving each breath over 1 second. The rationale is again to minimise time of interruption of chest compression.

Single shock strategy to defibrillation

The approach to defibrillation has also changed with a single shock of between 150j and 360j, depending on the equipment available.

It is felt that a resistant VF or VT that does not respond to a single shock is likely to be due to the myocardium being hypoxic.

Consequently the rapid restoration of good quality chest compressions are the priority, which should follow an unsuccessful attempt to defibrillate for a period of two minutes before defibrillation is attempted again.

Chapter 6 – Further reading

Chapter 6: Further Reading

Resuscitation Council (UK) Editorial Chair Jerry Nolan.	2005	Advanced Life Support Fifth Edition Resuscitation Council, London.
International Liaison Committee on Resuscitation. Part 4 Advanced Life Support 2005.	2005	International consensus on cardiopulmonary resuscitation and emergency cardiovascular care science with treatment recommendations Resuscitation 2005: 67:213-247.
International Liaison Committee on Resuscitation. Part 3 Defibrillation.	2005	International consensus on cardiopulmonary resuscitation and emergency cardiovascular care science with treatment recommendations 67:203-211.

Chapter 7

The 2005 paediatric and newborn resuscitation guidelines

The new guidelines for paediatric resuscitation and the resuscitation of the newborn were also published on 27 November 2005, with a plan to implement these new guidelines at the same time that the adult guidelines are to be implemented.

There is of course the consideration of change management taking time, particularly as some of the changes involve reconfiguration of machinery that is dependant on the resources outside the direct control of many healthcare providers.

It is planned for the distribution of adult related education materials to be in place by April 2006, with paediatric and neonatal following this. It has not been stated when child and neonatal educational material will be distributed. However, it is likely that many healthcare providers and Trusts will follow a staggered approach of implementation as inferred in the Resuscitation Council's literature in order to minimise the overhead of change management to resuscitation departments and services.

As with all changes within the new guidelines, there is recognition that there will be a period of overlap between the use of the old guidelines and the inclusion into practice of the new guidelines.

The Resuscitation Council recognises this likelihood and is keen for the clinician to acknowledge the value and appropriateness of previous guidelines when implementing the new, whilst always prioritising a consensus of approach in the practice environment.

What follows in this chapter is a faithful reproduction of the new guidelines in algorithm format as a quick reference guide for the busy clinician.

Chapter 7 Contents

The paediatric basic life support algorithm

Resuscitation Council (UK) 2005

Paediatric Basic Life Support

(Healthcare professionals
with a duty to respond)

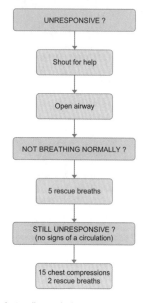

After 1 minute call resuscitation team then continue CPR

Paediatric FBAO treatment

Resuscitation Council (UK) 2005

Paediatric FBAO Treatment

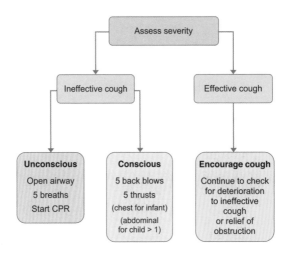

Paediatric advanced life support

Resuscitation Council (UK) 2005

Paediatric Advanced Life Support

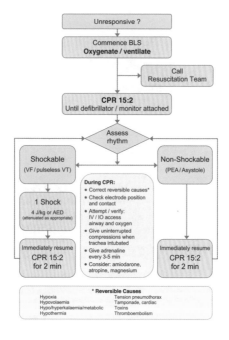

Newborn life support algorithm

Resuscitation Council (UK) 2005

Newborn Life Support

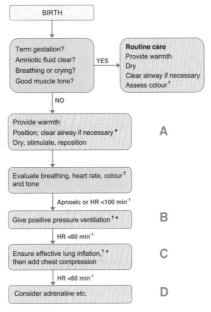

* Tracheal intubation may be considered at several steps
† Consider supplemental oxygen at any stage if cyanosis persists

Summary of key changes within the 2005 paediatric guidelines

- Children are either an infant up to one year old or a child from one year to puberty.

- There is no distinction between children above or below the age of 8.

- Single compression / ventilation ratio for all children.

- Assessment of breathing: Unresponsive and either not breathing or making agonal gasps.

- The rate and ratio of chest compressions has changed to 15:2 for the trained rescuer.

- The rate and ratio of chest compression s has changes to 30:2 for the untrained rescuer.

- An AED can be used for all children over one year of age.

- Single shock strategy to defibrillation of 4J/kg or AED, attenuated as appropriate.

- In the absence of a paediatric defibrillation capacity, an adult AED may be used.

Rationale for key changes within the 2005 paediatric guidelines

A key concern with the compilation of the new paediatric resuscitation guidelines was the application of the research findings that highlighted the fact many rescuers felt unable to rescue a child as they were not specifically trained and were therefore fearful of causing harm.

These guidelines have, where possible, attempted to make common many elements of both paediatric and adult guidelines in the knowledge that any intervention is likely to help.

As with the adult guidelines, attempts have been made to ease skill and knowledge retention through simplification of instruction.

Assessment of breathing

The designation not breathing normally has replaced the term and finding of not breathing.

It was identified by the Resuscitation Council that agonal breathing had not been previously identified and commencement of resuscitation was often in these instances delayed.

No distinction between children above or below the age of 8

The adoption of a single compression / ventilation ratio, along with the new advice of deploying AEDs at the early age of older than one year, means the guidelines are simpler in that no distinction is made at age 8 years.

30:2 ratio for the lay rescuer

The purpose of 30:2 ratio for the lay rescuer is again to enable the non-paediatric trained lay rescuer, and to also ensure simplicity of approach.

The AED if needed for the child can be used in children older than 8 years of age. However a modified attenuated manual or AED should be used in the one year to 8 year age group.

When paediatric defibrillation equipment is not available, the adult AED maybe used in children older than one year.

Chapter 7 – Further reading

Chapter 7: Further Reading

Resuscitation Council (UK) Editorial Chair Jerry Nolan.	2005	Advanced Life Support Fifth Edition Resuscitation Council, London.
International Liaison Committee on Resuscitation. Part 4 Advanced Life Support 2005.	2005	International consensus on cardiopulmonary resuscitation and emergency cardiovascular care science with treatment recommendations Resuscitation 2005: 67:213-247.
International Liaison Committee on Resuscitation. Part 3 Defibrillation	2005	International consensus on cardiopulmonary resuscitation and emergency cardiovascular care science with treatment recommendations 67:203-211.

Chapter 8

Medical emergencies

This chapter is intended to provide a resource for the clinician within all environments when encountering an emergency situation that needs a response that is swift, insightful specific and effective.

It provides key information on how to make a rapid assessment of what is the problem, what key interventions are needed, and in what order of priority.

Chapter 8 Contents

Chapter 8 Contents

First approach to the sick patient

When first approaching the patient in the circumstance of rapid and acute deterioration, the clinician should use a systematic approach with an incremental method to assess those areas that, if disrupted, represent the greatest risk to life.

The Resuscitation Council (UK) advocates the following approach:

A   AIRWAY

B   BREATHING

C   CIRCULATION

D   DISABILTY

E   EXPOSURE

This approach is discussed in this section.

AIRWAY

- Ensure that patient has a patent airway.

- Look listen feel, as described in Chapter 1.

- Secure airway if at all threatened using airway adjuncts, such as an oralpharengeal airway or, if necessary, intubation.

- Protect cervical spine with a jaw thrust if cervical injury suspected.

BREATHING

- Assess breathing: rate and efficiency.

- Bilateral air entry.

- Ausculate and percuss.

- Give oxygen if compromised.

CIRCULATION

- Palpation of carotid pulse.

- Look for signs of poor perfusion.

- Look for signs of shock.

- Look for signs of haemorrhage.

DISABILTY

- Does the patient have a known medical problem?

- Are there obvious signs such as the context of collapse?

- Are there relatives in attendance that can give a history?

- Assess level of consciousness using AVPU:

    - **A**lert

    - Responds to **V**oice

    - Responds to **P**ain

    - **U**nresponsive

EXPOSURE

- Undress the patient so a more thorough examination can be performed.

- Be mindful of the patient's risk to exposure and hypothermia.

M.O.V.E

When you arrive at the scene of an acutely deteriorated or peri-arrest patient within the healthcare environment, there are a number of actions that can be taken which will be of immediate benefit in second stage assessment and preparation for further deterioration if the patient proceeds to respiratory or cardiac arrest.

These actions, once embedded in the nurse's practice, can reduce anxiety, speed up management, assist the direction of others and ultimately may improve patient out come.

M = Monitor: Attach the patient to a cardiac monitor. If the patient collapses at this stage with no cardiac output, a greater range of management options are available to you, see VT/VF management under Chapter 3. Acquire and monitor vital observations, blood pressure, heart rate, oxygen saturations and respiratory rate.

O = Oxygen: Oxygen is indicated in most peri-arrest situations. Administer high flow oxygen. Caution should be given to patients who have, or are known to have, high arterial blood carbon dioxide levels. However, in life threatening hypoxia high flow oxygen is still given.

V = Venous access: A peri-arrest patient will need intravenous intervention of some kind and if the patient proceeds to cardiac arrest this procedure becomes more difficult. See Cannulation and venepuncture under Chapter 4.

E = ECG and Expert Help: A 12-lead electrocardiogram (ECG) is particularly useful in this situation if the collapse is a cardiac mediated event. The ECG can give valuable information about other problems such as electrolyte imbalance, see interpreting under Chapter 3. **Expert help must be summoned**. This may be by calling a medical emergency team, Cardiac Arrest team, or by fast bleeping a specific team member such as the anaesthetist or medical registrar.

Coma

Coma is where a patient is unrousable and unresponsive.

Management of coma:

- Secure airway if necessary

- Ensure breathing and circulation present

- Secure cervical spine

- M.O.V.E

Consider causes:

Hypoglycaemia – test and treat with 100ml of 20% glucose IV and repeat if necessary.

Opiate overdose – nalaxone 0.4mg IV every 2 minutes until respiration stable to a maximum of 2mg

Benzodiazepines – flumazenil 300 to 600 micrograms over 6 minutes

If fitting, treat with IV lorazepam 4mg in 1ml. If no IV access, use 10mg Diazepam per rectum.

Investigations:

- ABG, chest x-ray (CXR), examine chest. See Chapter 2

- FBC, U&Es, LFT, ESR

- Blood cultures, urine culture

- Drug levels. See chapter 5

- Toxicology screen

Having taken first line actions a secondary level assessment is needed to identify the cause of the coma and consolidate management. The cause will fall into metabolic or neurological category.

Metabolic

- Hypoxia, CO_2 narcosis (COPD)

- Septicaemia

- Hypothermia

- Hypoglycaemia, hyperglycaemia – ketoacidotic or hyperglycaemic hyperosmolar non-ketotic coma (HONK)

- Endocrine disruption – Addisonian crisis, Myxoedema

- Drugs, poisoning – alcohol, opiates, carbon monoxide

Neurological

- Trauma.

- Intra cerebral bleed:

    - Subarachnoid haematoma (SAH).

    - Subdural haematoma (SDH).

    - Cerebral vascular accident (CVA).

- Epilepsy – post-ictal.

- Infection – Meningitis, encephalitis, herpes.

- Tumour.

Consider the listed cause to guide your further investigations and management.

Acute Coronary Syndrome: Management of Acute Myocardial Infarction (AMI)

Acute myocardial infarction is most often caused by the rupture of an atherosclerotic plaque in a coronary artery. This causes the formation of a thrombus that blocks the artery, which in turns stops in from supplying blood to the territory of the heart that it supplies.

Myocardial Infarctions are most commonly described by which territory of the heart is affected, although every patient's coronary artery anatomy is individual to them, there are similarities amongst most patients' anatomies.

Territory is initially diagnosed by ECG, and then can be confirmed by an echocardiogram. The main territories of the heart, and the coronary arteries which may supply them are as follows:

- Anterior (Front and particularly the left ventricle)

    - Left Anterior Descending (LAD)

    - Left Main Stem (LMS)

    - LAD diagonals

- Inferior (Bottom)

    - Right Coronary Artery (RCA) in more than 70% of patients

    - Some patients – around 20% – have a dominant Circumflex artery

(CX) supplying the bottom of the heart

- Lateral (left side)

    - CX

    - LAD

    - LAD diagonals

- Posterior (back)

    - LMS

    - CX

Presentation of AMI

- The patient will appear distressed.

- Feeling of impending doom.

- Normally complaining of severe retrosternal chest pain or indigestion type pain, although diabetic patients are sometimes known not to report pain symptoms.

- Pain can radiate to arms, neck, throat, shoulders, or jaw.

- May have nausea or be vomiting.

- May be breathless.

- Tachycardia or bradycardic, depending on the location of the infarction.

- Blood pressure can be high, low or normal.

Initially:

- Monitor.
- Oxygen – caution with COPD.
- Venous access.
- 12-lead ECG.
- Bloods:
    - FBC.
    - Urea, Creatinine and Electrolytes.

> Troponin T peaks 12 hours after the event. A negative Troponin T, with no ECG changes, is a good indication of chest pain not caused by an acute myocardial infarction.

    - Lipid profile.
    - Cardiac Enzymes (CK, CK-MB).
    - Troponin T.

Assessment:

- History of pain / symptoms:
    - Description.
    - Severity.
    - Associated symptoms.
    - Onset.
    - Duration.
    - Trigger factors.
    - What relieves it?

- Past medical history.
- History of cardiac risk factors.
- Contraindications to thrombolysis.

Examination:

- BP.
- Pulse.
- JVP.
- Peripheral pulses.
- Capillary refill.
- Listen to heart sounds for murmurs.
- Examine chest for signs of heart failure.
- Chest x-ray.

Give:

- Aspirin 300mg dissolvable.
- Morphine 2.5 to 5mg IV.
- Metoclopramide 10mg IV.
- Glycerol Trinitrate (GTN) 2 puffs sublingually.
- Intravenous beta-blocker (e.g. Metoprolol).
- Consider DVT prophylaxis.

Thrombolysis reduces mortality if given as close to the AMI event as possible. The British Heart Foundation advises to aim to initiate Thrombolysis within 90 minutes of the event occurring ideally within 60 minutes.

Benefit can be seen in treatment given as late as 12 hours after the AMI event.

Indications for treatment with Thrombolysis require 2 or more of the following:

- ECG Ischemia:

    - S-T elevation greater than 2mm in 2 or more chest leads or S-T elevation greater than 1mm in 2 or more limb leads.

    - Posterior infarct. See chapter 3.

    - New onset left bundle branch block. See chapter 3.

- Troponin T rise of above 0.1.

- Definite history of ischemic pain and other symptoms.

Absolute contraindications for treatment with Thrombolysis:

- Previous hemorrhagic stroke at any time.

- Other strokes or cerebrovascular events, within one year.

- Known intracranial neoplasm.

- Active internal bleeding (except menses).

- Suspected aortic dissection.

- Acute pericarditis.

Streptokinase and Tissue Plasminogen Activator (TPA) are the most commonly used thrombolytic agents:

- Streptokinase:

    - Dose 1.5 million units in 100ml of normal saline IV over 1 hour.

- If hypotension occurs slow infusion rate.

- Watch for signs of haemorrhage.

Acute Coronary Syndrome: Management of unstable angina

Unstable angina is a term with different meanings attributed to it and more frequently it is being described within the collective term of acute coronary syndromes. However in terms of management it can be described as angina occurring at rest, or minimal exertion and is associated with a greater risk of myocardial infarction.

The cause is most commonly plaque disruption and the subsequent development of intraluminal thrombus formation. This does not completely occlude the artery as in an AMI, and depending on whether a rise in Troponin is evident, it is described as unstable angina or non-Q wave infarction.

Investigations:

• Take ECG at time of pain.

• Serial ECGs.

• ECG may show S-T depression. See Chapter 3.

• Flat or inverted "T" waves.

Blood tests:

- Troponin T.
- FBC.
- Urea.
- Creatinine and electrolytes.
- Glucose.
- Fasting lipids.
- Cardiac enzymes.

Examine:

- Pulse.
- Heart sounds.
- Chest auscultation.
- JVP.

Heart failure is a common complication and may warrant a more expansive management plan intervention.

- M.O.V.E
- Place patient in monitored environment preferably CCU or acute medical environment with cardiology capacity.
- Analgesia – Diamorphine 2.5 - 5mg IV
- Metoclopramide 10mg IV
- Nitrates GTN spray 400mcg x 2
- Sublingual GTN tablets 500mg x 2
- Aspirin 300mgs PO, unless contraindicated

Beta blockers

- Metoprolol 50-100mgs 8 hourly **or**

- Atenolol 50 -100mgs in 24 hours.

Beta blockers are contraindicated in asthma, COPD, LVF and coronary artery spasm, in which case give calcium antagonist:

- Verapamil 80-120mgs 8 hourly PO or

- Diltiazem 60-120mgs 8 hourly PO.

Heparinise with low molecular weight heparin:

- Enoxaparin 1mg per kg 12 hourly.

Pulmonary oedema management

The causes of pulmonary oedema are varied but can often be related to cardiovascular disease. Causes include:

- Left ventricular heart failure following myocardial infarction or ischemic heart disease.
- Mitral value stenosis.
- Malignant hypertension.
- Fluid overload.
- Renal failure.
- In adequate dialysis in the chronic renal failure patient.
- Acute Respiratory Distress Syndrome (ARDS).

Presentation:

- The patient will appear distressed and can have a feeling of impending doom
- Breathless
- Raised Jugular Venous Pressure (JVP)
- Bilateral inspiratory crackles on chest auscultation
- Hypertension
- Tachycardia
- CXR will show diffuse whiteness opacity with indistinct costophrenic margins, and often shows cardiomegaly.

Note: In ARDS, unless the patient has IHD heart size may be normal.

- Sit the patient upright in bed.

- M.O.V.E.

Exercise caution when giving oxygen to chronic CO_2 retaining patients, such as COPD. If high CO_2 is acute, marked by a low or normal HCO_3, and is likely to be related to the pulmonary oedema, then high flow oxygen is normally safe to administer alongside other treatment.

- Diamorphine 2.5mg to 5mg.

- Furosemide 40 - 80mg IV.

- GTN 2 puffs or Sub-lingual GTN 300 mg. Do not give if systolic BP below 90mmHg.

- Nitrate infusion if BP has a systolic of 100mm Hg or above.

- Typically isosorbide dinitrate 2 to 8mg IVI titrated against any fall in blood pressure.

If patient does not improve give further Furosemide 40 to 80mg IV. Alternatively consider continuous positive airway pressure (CPAP) in place of incremental diuretic therapy.

Cardiogenic shock

- M.O.V.E.

- Move to a critical care environment such as CCU, HDU or ITU as soon as possible.

- Diamorphine 2.5mg to 5 mg IV for the pain and anxiety.

Bloods:

- Urea.

- Creatine and Electrolytes.

- CK.

- Troponin T.

- FBC.

- LFTs.

- Coagulation screen.

Correct any electrolyte imbalance.

Chest x-ray – look for tension pneumothorax, aortic dissection tamponade, pulmonary congestion.

ABG – see Chapter 2.

Correct acid base balance

- Serial ECG

- Central Venous Pressure line measurements

- Optimize filling pressure

- Consider plasma expander such as gelufusine

- Consider inotopic support

- Consider intra-aortic balloon pump

Acute severe asthma

Assessment	
Severe asthma:	Life threatening asthma:
• Unable to complete sentences	• Peak flow < 33% of predicted best
• Respiratory rate >25/minute	• Silent chest
• Pulse rate >110/minute	• Cyanosis
• Peak flow <50% of predicted best	• Feeble respiratory effort
	• Exhaustion / coma
	• Confusion
	• Bradycardia
	Arterial blood gases: PCO_2 > 5kPa PO_2 <8kPa pH <7.35

M – Monitor oxygen saturation, peak flow and ABGs

O – Oxygen 100% via re-breath bag

V – Venous access

E – ECG monitoring is of value in life threatening circumstance even though not cardiac mediated.

E for Expert help – An anesthetist or medical emergency team will be probably be required

- Assess severity of attack,

Illicit anesthetic help ITU and MET support if life threatening (Medical Emergency Team)

- Sit patient upright

- Give Oxygen 100% via re-breath bag

- Salbutamol 5mgs nebulized with Oxygen

- Hydrocortisone 200mgs IV or 30mgs of prednisolone

- Chest x-ray to exclude pnemothorax

- ECG to assist exclusion of cardiac cause and pulmonary embolism

- Bloods:

    - D-Dimer to exclude pulmonary embolism

    - Urea

    - Creatinine and Electrolytes

    - FBC

    - Theophylline levels

In life threatening

- Ipratropium 0.5mg with the nebulized Salbutamol

- Aminophylline 5mg per kg IV bolus over 20 minutes

- Consider Salbutamol intravenous infusion

- Consider intravenous infusion of Magnesium Sulphate

> If the patient is currently taking oral theophtllines then omit this bolus but ensure serum level is at therapeutic range

If no improvement:

- Continue with 100% oxygen therapy

- Nebulized Salbutamol every 15 minutes

- Continue with Ipratropium 0.5mg every 6 hours

- Consider ICU referral

COPD – Chronic Obstructive Pulmonary Disease

- Oxygen therapy starting at 24%

Caution with CO_2 retainers as oxygen lack is often the stimulation to respiration in this chronic pathology and radically increasing oxygen levels can have the effect of reducing the respiration rate and causing apnea.

- ABGs – See Chapter 2

Aim for PaO_2 of > 8.0kPa

PCO_2 to fall by 1.5kPa

- Nebulized Salbutamol 5mgs 4 hourly
- Ipratropium 0.5mg 6 hourly
- IV hydrocortisone 200mg and oral prednisolone 30mg

Examine chest – See Chapter 2

Chest x-ray – See Chapter 2

Look for signs of infection: also check no signs of pnemothorax or pulmonary embolism.

- Treat with antibiotics.

- Typically amoxicillin 500mg four times daily if penicillin allergy excluded.

- If pH < 7.26 and pCO_2 is rising referral on for more in progressive respiratory management.

NIPPV Non invasive positive pressure ventilation

This is the treatment of choice as it rests tired muscles of respiration while improving pO_2 and pCO_2 levels whilst avoiding the complications of endotracheal ventilation.

Intubation and ventilation

It is often difficult to wean COPD patients from ventilation once initiated and they are more prone to complication of ventilation.

The decision to ventilate will depend on the patients quality of life which is best gained on admission in conjunction with relatives if available.

It is difficult making this decision in an acute situation without access to the patient's wants and pre-morbid status.

Respiratory stimulant such as doxapram

Less frequently used, this drug is considered a short term adjunct while awaiting ventilation.

Side effects confusion, agitation, nausea and tachycardia.

Tension pneumothorax

This is a medical emergency that will result in cardiac arrest if not promptly treated.

Presentation:

- Respiratory distress.
- Tachycardia.
- Hypotension.
- Distended neck veins.
- Tracheal deviation away from the side of the pneumothorax.
- Hyper resonate lung on percussion of the affected side.
- Reduced breath sounds on the affected side.

Management:

- Immediate needle thoracocentesis.
- M.O.V.E.
- Ensure pulse oxygemeitry is also in place.

Needle thoracocentesis procedure

- Position the patient in 45 degree, sitting position.
- Palpate landmark – the upper border of the third rib in the midclavicular line, second intercostal space.
- Attach a 5ml syringe to a large bore cannula (Brown or Orange - 14g)

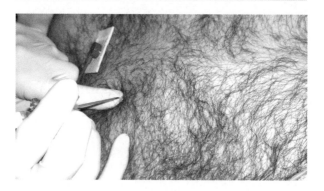

- Attach a 3-way tap.

- Puncture the skin at the level of above landmark.

- Carefully insert the needle at a slightly downwards angle into the pleural space while aspirating the syringe.

- In tension pneumothorax, often you will hear a pop or feel a change of resistance.

- Withdraw the needle while gently advancing the cannula downwards into position.

- Secure cannula.

- Drain until no further drainage or to a maximum of 30ml per kg (to a maximum of 2.5 litres).

- Follow up with insertion of a chest drain, following primary survey and management.

Gastric intestinal bleed and shock

- Manage reduced consciousness and, if necessary A.B.C.

- M.O.V.E

- Insert a large bore (14 - 16g) cannula into both arms, use ante cubital site. See Chapter 4.

Bloods:

- Group and Save and Cross match 6 units

- FBC

- Clotting screen

- U&Es and LFTs

- Glucose

Infuse with large volume of plasma expander, typically 1 litre of Gelofusin. If not available administer any fluid such as normal saline.

If patient remains shocked give blood O Rh negative until cross match specific blood is available.

- Correct clotting abnormalities.

- Secure central vascular access.

- Monitor fluid balance and urine output, catheterise.

- Arrange endoscopic investigations for diagnosis and management.

Management of status epilepticus

- Protect airway.
- If airway is at risk and airway adjuncts are needed take caution with insertion.
- Recovery position.
- Oxygen therapy at 100%.
- IV access.
- Test blood sugar with BM test.
- Give dextrose 100ml of 20% if needed.
- Give Thiamine 250mg IV or a pair of Pabrinx ampoules (vitamins B&C) if alcoholism suspected to avoid Wernickes encephalopathy complications.

Bloods:

- Anticonvulsant levels if indicated
- U&Es
- LFT
- FBC

> Give Lorazepam 4mgs slow IV bolus or Diazepam 10mgs PR if no IV access available. If seizures continue give IV phenytoin 15mg per kg at a rate not exceeding 50mg per minute.

If the seizures continue call for anaesthetic support. If 20 minutes have elapsed before control achieved refer to anaesthetics.

Management of hypoglycaemia

Presentation:

- Agitation

- Confusion

- Aggression

- Sweating

- Collapse

In a first contact environment such as Accident and Emergency, the patient's history is not always known and this presentation can be wrongly attributed to alcohol.

- Make a diagnosis on BM blood sugar.

- Ensure patient is not a known alcoholic or malnourished.

- Secure IV access.

- Give IV dextrose 50% 50ml.

- If not response after the first dose repeat.

- If IV access is problematic use Glucagon Img IM.

- Follow up in controlled environment with diabetic care referral.

Diabetic ketoacidosis

Presentation:

- This can only occur with type 1 diabetic (DM)
- Usually a 2-3 day history of gradual decline with:

    - Polyuria.
    - Polydipsia.
    - Anorexia.
    - Dehydration.
    - Vomiting.
    - Abdominal pain.
    - Loss of appetite.
    - Lethargy.
    - May present as coma.

Common preceded events:

- Infection.
- Surgery.
- Myocardial infarctions
- Non-compliant patient.
- Wrongly prescribed insulin.

Diagnosis is made on the presence of ketosis and acidosis with a pH of less than 7.3.

IV access and commence intravenous fluids immediately.
Regime of replacement:

- 1,000 0.9% normal saline stat
- 1,000 0.9% normal saline over next hour
- 1,000 0.9% normal saline over next 2 hours
- 1,000 0.9% normal saline over next 4 hours
- 1,000 0.9% normal saline over next 6 hours

Give insulin 10u actrapid if blood sugar levels > 20 mmol/L.
Investigations:

- Blood glucose.
- U&Es.
- HCO_3 osmolarity.
- ABGs.
- FBC.
- Blood culture.
- Test urine for ketones.
- MSU.
- Chest x-ray.
- Insulin sliding scale
- Add potassium to on-going fluid replacement titrated to serum levels
- Hourly glucose, U&Es, HCO_3
- Monitor fluid balance, use urinary catheter if necessary.

- If management protracted central access should be sought.

Insulin sliding scale

Make insulin solution 50u actrapid to a gross volume of 50ml made with 0.9% normal saline

- 50u to 50mls

Blood glucose level	Actrapid insulin	In infection or insulin resistance
4.0-7.9	1ml / hr	2 ml / hr
8.0-11.9	2ml / hr	4 ml / hr
12.0-16.0	3ml / hr	6 ml / hr
>16.0	4ml / hr	8 ml / hr

Potassium will move into body tissue with treatment therefore hourly U&Es are need to guide K+ for the following regimen.

Serum K+	KCL to be added to each litre of fluid
<3.0mmols	40mmols
<4.0mmols	30mmols
<5.0mmols	20mmols

Hyperglycaemic Hyperosmolar Non-ketotic Coma (HONK)

- Affects non-insulin diabetic only

- Patients are invariably old

- A week or more history of feeling increasingly unwell:

    - Polyuria

    - Polydipsia

    - Dehydration

    - Vomiting

    - May present in coma.

- Marked dehydration

- Elevated glucose greater than 35mmols per litre

- No ketones as the patient has not switched to ketone metabolism, for the same reason acidosis is also absent.

- Osmolarity is greater than 340mosmol/kg

Management of HONK

Hyperosmolarity of the blood will increase the risk of DVT therefore give prophylactic heparin.

Rehydrate with 0.9% normal saline.

Regime of replacement:

- 500 0.9% normal saline stat

- 1,000 0.9% normal saline over next 2 hours

- 1,000 0.9% normal saline over next 4 hours

- 1,000 0.9% normal saline over next 8 hours

Exercise caution with large volumes of fluid IV with the elderly.

Insulin may not be needed but add to regime only if other management is proving insufficient.

Give insulin in low doses titrated to effect.

Monitor serum and replace potassium particularly in the presence of insulin use.

Acute renal failure

- Acute onset over hours or days.
- Oliguria, anuria or polyuria dependent on cause.
- May have pulmonary oedema.
- Systemic oedema a may be present.
- Bloods will show elevated urea and creatinine and potentially Potassium levels.

Acute renal failure (ARF) may occur as the primary illness or more commonly as a complication of severe disruption of some other bodily system such as sepsis, following surgery or trauma.

Causes:

- Acute tubular necrosis (ATN) most commonly associated with circulatory collapse.
- Nephrotoxic agents such as:
    - NSAIDs.
    - Aminoglycosides.
    - Amphotericin B.
    - Tetracyclines.
    - ACE inhibitors.
- Rhabdomyolysis.
- Obstruction.
- Hepatorenal syndrome.

Management of Acute Renal Failure (ARF)

- M.O.V.E. Remove previous access if sepsis considered the cause and no locus identified.
- Monitor urine output – Catheterise and measure urine output hourly.
- Bloods:
    - U&Es.
    - FBC.
    - LFTs.
    - Hepatitis serology.
    - Autoantibodies.
    - Blood cultures.
- Chest x-ray for pulmonary oedema and heart enlargement.
- ECG for tented or peaked "T" waves due to Hyperkalaemia.
- Also observe for ectopic beats on an ECG monitor or 12-lead ECG.
- Renal tract ultrasound and KUB looking for obstructive cause.
- Urine: Dip sticks for protein and blood.
- Urine microscopy

White cell cast = possible infective cause

Red cell casts = possible inflammatory glomeruli cause

- Manage hyperkalaemia if present
- Fluid assessment. See ARF appendix.
- Treat oliguria with low intravascular volume with fluid challenge.

Fluid challenge = 250 to 500ml of colloid or normal saline over 30 minutes.

- Give second fluid challenge if first proves ineffective.

Take care with bolus volumes of fluid in the petit, frail, and elderly and with a strong cardiac history. Titrate volumes accordingly.

- If oliguria persists consider:
    - Furosemide
    - Renal dose dopamine 2 to 5 micrograms per kg per minute
- If volume overloaded consider haemodialysis and haemo filtration.

- Manage acidosis with bicarbonate infusion 50ml of 8.4% sodium bicarbonate.
- Refer patient to a renal physician or renal unit.

Fluid balance assessment

Collect data:

• Fluid balance if previously recorded.

• Hourly volumes of urine voided.

• Weight change if known.

Physical signs:

Skin turgor – Take a pinch of skin between finger and thumb gentle twist and release then watch the skin return to its natural position.

A swift return suggests elastic properties to the skin which could be interpreted as containing an appropriate or high volume of interstitial fluid. This is more difficult to assess in the elderly and may not be an accurate assessment.

Jugular venous pressure (JVP): High JVP shows a loaded venous system, whereas not visible may indicate low venous pressure and may be low volume related.

Central venous pressure (CVP): Consistently raised CVP measurements are likely to suggest overload. Note that right sided heart failure, high respiratory pressures, pulmonary valve stenosis and tricuspid regurgitation can also cause high CVP.

Signs of systemic oedema, in the legs if the patient is ambulatory and in the sacral area if bed bound.

Signs of pulmonary oedema:

- Chest x-ray for signs of pulmonary oedema
- Examine chest for signs of pulmonary oedema. See Chapter 2.

Blood pressure, and pulse: Note postural changes.

Assess the patients serum protein, particularly albumin and note a low Hb.

The fluid assessment will enable you understand where the fluid is and plan treatment accordingly.

Elevated Intravascular volume	Interissual Fluid
• Possible BP elevation	• May have systemic oedema
• Possible JVP elevated	• BP maybe low
• Possible CVP elevated	• May have postural drop
• May have pulmonary oedema	• CVP maybe low
	• JVP maybe not visible and therefore possible low
	• Albumin maybe low
	• May have olguria
	Albumin (35-50gm/litre)

Management of Hyperkalaemia

Hyperkalaemia (Elevated potassium) is a life threatening condition and, if untreated, can lead to ventricular fibrillation. See Chapter 1.

A potassium level of greater than 6.5mmols/l will need emergency management.

However, there are instances when potassium of this level is routinely seen in the chronic renal dialysis patient immediately prior to the next treatment.

Causes include: Renal failure, ACE inhibitors, potassium sparing diuretics, overdose of potassium supplements.

ECG changes:

- Tall tented "T" waves

- May have flattening "P" waves

- May have increasing P-R intervals

- Widening of QRS complex

Treatment:

- Insulin and dextrose

- 15-20 IU Actrapid with 50ml 50% Glucose

- Calcium Gluconate 10ml of 10% IV then Calcium resonium 15gm 3 to 4 times a day

- Dialysis

Anaphylaxis

Presentation:

- History of contact with a likely allergen
- Skin changes:
    - Urticaria
    - Rash
    - Erythema
    - Itching particularly local to the point of contact
- Respiratory signs:
    - Dyspnea
    - Wheeze
    - Angioedema
    - Stridor
- Cardiovascular signs
    - Tachycardia
    - Hypotension
    - Cardiac arrhythmias
    - Sudden collapse
- Further signs:
    - Feeling of impending doom
    - Shock
    - Collapse

- Further presentation:

    - Nausea

    - Vomiting

    - Abdominal pain

    - Diarrhoea

    - Agitation or confusion

    - Tremor

    - Cool to the touch – peripherally shut down

    - Localised effect

Remember anaphylaxis may and often presents in atypical fashion.

History is of particular value, particularly a history of allergen contact.

Similarly a history of previous allergic response of lesser magnitude that could point to a chronology of previous sensitisation.

Anaphylactoid is a reaction of similar pathophysiology but does not reflect sensitisation to a particular antigen. For purposes of acute management this can and should be treated the same as anaphylaxis.

Management:

- Adrenaline 500mcgs I/M

- Chlorphenamine 10 to 20mgs I/V or I/M

- 1 litre of normal saline (0.9%) or a plasma expander such as Gelofusin over 30 minutes (Give with caution if the patient is elderly has concurrent cardiac problems or other issues of vulnerability)

- Hydrocortisone 100 to 200mg I/M or I/V

- Consider Salbutamol 5mg nebuliser

Chapter 8 – Further reading

Chapter 8: Further Reading

International Liaison Committee on Resuscitation	2005	Acute coronary syndromes: emergency cardiovascular care science with treatment recommendations Resuscitation 2005:67:248-269
Bertrand M E et al	2002	Management of acute coronary syndromes presenting without persistent ST segment elevation European heart journal 23:1809-1840
European Society of Cardiology	2004	Management of acute myocardial infarction presenting with ST segment elevation European heart journal 24:28-66
Fox K A et al	2004	British cardiac working group on the definition of myocardial infarction Heart 90:603-609
Blomstrom-Lundqvist et al	2003	Guidelines for the management of the patient with supraventricular arrhythmias European heart journal24: 1857-1897
Barbara B	1995	A Guide to physical examination and history taking Sixth Edition Lippincott London

Chapter 8: Further Reading

Mahoney B, Smith W	2005	Emergency interventions for hyperkalaemia Cochrane database system review CD 003235
British Thoracic Society	2003	British guidelines on the management of asthma Thorax 58(Supp 1): 1-94
Mertes PM, Laxenaire	2003	Anaphylactic and anaphylactoid reactions occurring during anaesthesia in France in 1999-2000 Anaesthesiology 99:536-545
Joint working party association of anaesthetists	2003	Suspected Anaphylactic reactions associated with anaesthesia British society for allergy & immunology 3rd Ed
British Thoracic Society	2002	Non invasive ventilation in acute respiratory failure Thorax 57(3): 192-211
Keenan S Sinuff T et al	2003	Chronic obstructive pulmonary disease: a systematic review of the literature Annals of internal medicine138, 861-870
Stroller JK	2003	Acute exacerbations of chronic obstructive pulmonary disease New England Journal of medicine346, 988-994
Beaman M Adu	1992	Acute renal failure Care of the critical ill patient pp515-530 Berlin Springer

Chapter 8: Further Reading

Blakey S Smith G	2003	Acute renal failure and replacement therapy in the ICU Anaesthetics & intensive care medicine 108 111
Holly L T, Kelly D F et al	2002	Cervical spine trauma associated with severe head injury Journal of neurosurgery 96(3), 285- 91
Lawn n D, Wijdicks E F M	2002	Status epilepticus: a critical review of management options Canadian journal of neurological science
Maas A I R Dearden M Teasdale G M et al	1997	EBIC guidelines for the management of severe head injury in adults Acta neurochirurgia (Wien) 139, 286- 294
Rees G Shah S Hanley C et al	2002	Subarachnoid haemorrhage a clinical overview Nursing standard 16(42) 47-56
Aviles R J, Aaskari A T et al	2002	Troponin levels in patients with acute coronary syndrome New England journal of medicine 346,2047-2052
Smith G, Poplett N	2002	Knowledge of acute aspects of care in junior doctors Post graduate medical journal 78, 335-338
	2004	Oxford text book of medicine Churchill Livingston London

Chapter 8: Further Reading

Cooper N, Cramp P	2003	Essential guide to acute care BMJ Books London

Chapter 9

Surgical management

Surgery is a specialist function that generates a lot of activity and interest for the clinician outside of the theatre environment, what follows in this chapter is a description of some of the more common issues that arise with the surgical patient and for the management of the surgical patient.

Chapter 9 Contents

Surgical emergencies: The acute abdomen

Acute presentation
Unwell
Signs and symptoms within abdomen

Look for signs of shock:

- Low blood pressure.

- Postural drop in blood pressure.

- Tachycardia.

- Peripherally shut down.

- Poor capillary refill.

Look for signs of Peritonitis:

- Shock.

- Lying still.

- Abdominal pain on coughing.

- Tenderness.

- Rebound.

- Board Like abdominal rigidity.

- Absence of bowel sounds.

- Possible gas under diagram on chest x-ray.

Possible causes:

- Rupture of internal organ.

- Spleen, aorta, ectopic pregnancy, history of trauma, particularly blunt trauma.

Possible causes of peritonitis:

- Perforation of:

- Duodenal ulcer

- Peptic ulcer

- Appendix

- Diverticulum

- Bowel

- Gall bladder.

Surgical emergencies: Preparation for emergency surgery

Consider the urgency for surgery. In extreme haemorrhage the patient may have to go straight to theatre however if there is time:

- Make patient NBM.
- Contact the surgical team.
- Inset a large bore intravenous cannula (16 to 18g) in case the need arises to administer quick fluids in shock.
- Manage shock with fluid replacement therapy 0.9% normal saline unless excess blood is being lost.
- Control pain.
- Obtain consent.
- Consider other medical history and make provision e.g. diabetes mellitus.
- Give prophylactic IV antibiotics.
- Carry out:
    - ECG.
    - Chest x-ray.
- Blood tests:
    - FBC.
    - Group, save and cross match at least 4 units.
    - U&Es.
    - LFTs.

- Clotting studies.

- Blood cultures.

Bowel obstruction

Presentation:

- Nausea and vomiting.

- Colicky abdominal pain.

- Distension.

- Altered bowel habit. Can have absolute constipation with no wind being passed.

High obstruction tinkling bowel sounds may be heard.

Bowel sounds may be absent

Further test:

- Abdominal x-ray may show excess gas in dilated loop of gut.

- Excessive fluid levels on erect film.

Management:

- If strangulated gut then urgent surgery is indicated.

Otherwise:

"Drip and Suck"

- Pass naso-gastric tube and allow free drainage.

- Insert an IV cannula and administer fluid to hydrate.

The abdominal examination

First glance assessment:

- Does the patient look pale and shocked?
- Is the patient lying rigidly as though suffering with extreme pain?

History:

- Where is the pain?
- Type of pain?
- What relieves the pain?
- How long has this been a problem?
- Other symptoms such as nausea and vomiting?
- Are there altered bowel habits?

System signs:

- Distension
- Ascites
- Spider naevi. Dilated arterioles causing a minute red papule in the skin, the small branching vessels resembling spider legs. This is a sign of liver disease.
- Jaundice
- Venous engorgement

Abdominal examination:

- On palpation does the pain worsen?
- Where is the pain located?

The abdomen

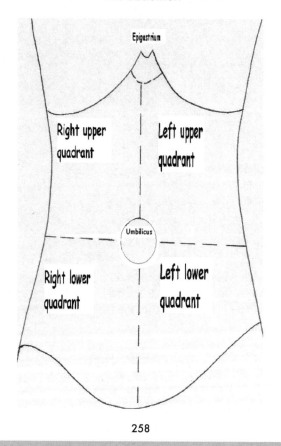

Epigastrium

Myocardial infarction
Peptic ulcer
Acute cholecysititis
Perforated oesophagus

Right upper quadrant

Acute cholecysititis
Duodenal ulcer
Hepatitis
Hepatomegaly
Pyelonephritis
Appendicitis

Left upper quadrant

Ruptured spleen
Gastric ulcer
Aortic aneurysm
Perforated colon
Pyelonephritis

Umbilicus

Intestinal obstruction

Acute pancreatitis

Early appendicitis

Mesenteric thrombus

Aortic aneurysm

Diverticulitis

Right lower quadrant

Appendicitis

Salpingitis

Tubo-ovarian abscess

Ruptured ectopic pregnancy

Incarcerated hernia

Mesenteric adenitis

Crohns disease

Perforated caecum

Left lower quadrant

Sigmoid diverticulitis

Tubo-ovarian abscess

Ruptured ectopic pregnancy

Incarcerated hernia

Crohns disease

Ulcerative colitis

Crohns disease

Pre-operative clerking check list

The purpose of the pre-operative clerking is to:

- Ensure the right person goes for surgery. Check with the patient's identity and ensure it corresponds with the name band they are wearing.

- Ensure that the correct procedure is performed.

- Through the process of clerking check that the operation is still clinical appropriate.

- Reduce risks of surgery/consider other therapeutic options.

- Ensure that the patient is optimised for surgery. Surgery has inherent risks which to some extent are known and planned for. What furthers the risk of surgery at the level of the individual is the vulnerability of the patient relative to the presence of other diseases.

- Achieve informed consent from the patient. Make sure the patient understands the implications of having and not having surgery, any possible complications and the likely success rate.

History of presenting complaint:

- Past medical history

- Known allergies. Highlight on the patient's notes, drug chart and computer record.

- Current medications.

- Social history.

- Examination, pertinent to the known problem.

It is often of value to draw a picture of lesions or morbid changes in organ structures relative to the presenting illness as an accurate record at a specific point in time. A photograph, if available, is also valuable.

Systemic examination:

- Cardiovascular.

- Respiratory.

- Neurological.

- Renal.

- Endocrine.

- Others as appropriate.

This element is essential in identifying risk of surgery.

Pre-operative clerking

Blood tests

- U&Es.

- FBC.

- Group and save / Group and cross match units depending on type of surgery.

- Coagulation screen.

- Glucose pin prick test (BM stix).

- LFT if history of jaundice or liver disease.

- C- Reactive Protein (CRP).

- Test therapeutic levels in blood of drugs such as digoxin.

Other tests:

- ECG if over 60 or known to have been / are at risk of cardiac problems.

- CXR if over 60 or known to have been / are at risk of respiratory problems.

Specific concerns for the diabetic patient:

- Ensure blood glucose level is known.

- Achieve control pre-operatively using dextrose and insulin infusions (sliding scale).

Specific concerns for Coagulopathy or therapeutic anti-coagulation:

- Ensure clotting studies are available well in advance pre operatively.

- Seek advice on reducing dose of anti coagulates.

- Avoid epidurals, spinal and regional blocks.

Post-operative care

Hypotension and shock

- Tilt head of bed down

- Give oxygen

- Ensure large bore cannula (14-16g) is in place. 2 are ideal.

- Cardiac monitor if likely to deteriorate further.

- Restore volume with fluids.

- If the cause is bleeding restore with blood or colloid plasma expander until blood arrives.

Hypotension due to Hypovolaemia

Fluid balance assessment

- Check input/output records

- Check JVP

- CVP

- Blood pressure relative to pre-operative recording

- Heart rate

- Skin turgor

- Urine concentration

Restore volume by increasing IV infusion rate.

Pyrexia post operatively in the first 24 hours is not uncommon and often relates to lung collapse at the time of surgery.

Treat with physiotherapy and early mobilisation.

Pyrexia beyond 24 hours or high temperature should prompt an infection screen:

- Examine chest
- Wound site
- Signs of peritonism
- Urinary Tract Infection (UTI)
- Signs of DVT
- Signs of mennigism

Send blood cultures

- Shortness of breath post operatively:
- Sit up
- Give oxygen (Caution in CO_2 retentive)
- ABGs
- Chest x-ray
- Look for signs of pulmonary oedema
- Look for signs pnemothorax
- Look for signs of atelectasis

Treat findings

Has not passed urine (HNPU):

- Ensure blood pressure is within accepted limits to adequately perfuse the kidneys. Mean ABP between 60 - 120mm of mercury.

- Examine patient for palpable bladder, urinary retention is not uncommon.

- Check patency of urinary catheter if in place, and consider bladder washout or irrigation.

- Check fluid balance as described previously.

- Check urea, creatinine, and electrolyte levels.

- If renal failure suspected refer on to nephrologists.

Chapter 9 – Further reading

Chapter 9: Further Reading		
National Blood Users Group	2001	A guideline for transfusion of red blood cells in surgical patients
Howe J R	1983	Manual of patient care in neurosurgery Little brown & Co Boston/Toronto
Marieb E M	2001	Human anatomy and physiology Benjamin Cummings San Francisco
Alexander M, Fawcett J, Runciman P J (Eds)	2002	Nursing practice Hospital and home: The adult Churchill Livingston London
Mellor S	1999	Recent advances in surgery Churchill Livingston London

Chapter 10

The neurological system and neurological emergencies

The neurological system is affected by any systemic illness. It is the neurological system that we in healthcare work hardest to protect, as a neurological insult can be life terminating or cause a dramatic fall in the quality of life of the patient.

What follows in this chapter is an overview of the nature of presenting neurological illness and management for the more common neurological emergencies.

Chapter 10 Contents

Raised intracranial pressure (ICP)

Raised ICP constitutes a medical emergency as the nature of the non-compliant box of the skull does not allow for changes in pressure and volume of the brain and tissue of adjacent structures.

Rapid onset of detrimental neurological symptoms will follow if this situation remains unresolved. Raised ICP relative to oedema has three source mechanisms:

- Vasogenic – increased vaso permeability due to tumour, trauma, ischcaemia and infection.

- Cytotoxic – cell death from hypoxia.

- Interstitial – for example obstructive hydrocephalus.

Causes:

- Tumour

- Head injury

- Menigoencephalitis

- Brain abscess

- Hydrocephalus

- Cerebral oedema

- Haemorrhage – Subdural, Extradural, Subarachnoid, Intracerebral, Intraventricular

Raised intracranial pressure: Presentation

- Headache

- Drowsiness

- Vomiting

- Seizures

- Restlessness

- Reduced level of consciousness

- Irritability

- Falling pulse

- Raising B/P

- Coma

- Cheyne-stoke respiration

- Pupils constricted initially then dilated at later stage

- Investigations:

- Blood cultures:

- FBC

- U&E

- CRP

- Glucose

- Clotting screen

- Serum osmolarity

- Chest x-ray

- CT or MRI scan of head

- Lumber puncture if safe. Caution lumber puncture where there is a discrepancy of pressure across the CSF system can cause coning.

- Contraindicated in intracranial mass lesion.

- Trauma.

- Focal signs.

- Coagulopathy.

- Middle ear pathology.

- Papilloedema.

Management of raised ICP

The management intent is to reduce the ICP:

- Manage ABC.

- Treat hypotension associated with ICP.

- Define cause.

- Elevate bed head.

- Intubate and hyperventilate in order to lower pCO_2 which will cause vasoconstriction which is very effective at reducing ICP.

- Osmotic agents are of some value in short term management:

    - Mannitol 20% solution at 5ml/L over 20 minutes.

    - Dexamethasone 10mgs IV is useful with raised ICP secondary to oedema around tumours: Followed by 4mg at 6 hours.

- Manage in intensive environment

- Treat cause

Head injury

- Assess patient using GCS (gold standard in most centres)

- Look for equal pupils with a brisk reaction to light (Good tug)

- Unequal pupils evident of third cranial nerve palsy

Glasgow Coma Score (GCS)		
Eye opening (E)	Verbal response (V)	Motor Response (M)
4 = Spontaneous	5 = Normal conversation	6 = Normal
3 = To voice	4 = Disoriented conversation	5 = Localises to pain
2 = To pain	3 = Words but not coherent	4 = Withdraws to pain
1 = None	2 = No words, only sounds	3 = Decorticate posture
	1 = None	2 = Decerebrate
		1 = None
Total = E + V + M		

- Level of consciousness

- BP

- Pulse

- Observe for hemiplegia or weakness

Involve neurosurgeon as early as possible, particularly if third cranial nerve palsy evident.

- **A**irway and cervical spine (stabilise), **B**reathing and **C**irculation

- Monitor

- Oxygen

- Secure airway – intubate and ventilate, if necessary

- Manage shock, if necessary

- Stop bleeding and treat lost volume is the common management. However, the argument continues regarding "to give or not give" fluids in trauma.

- Manage seizures with lorazepam or diazepam

- ABG, glucose, FBS, Blood alcohol, toxology screen, clotting studies

- Neuro examination

- Secondary survey

- Examine any skull lacerations looking for step deformity

- Look for CSF leak at nose or ears

- CT head and C spine

- Chest x-ray

Meningitis

Meningitis is an emergency, particularly meningococcal meningitis which is a condition that is very rapidly progressive.

Presentation:

- Headache

- Neck stiffness

- Photophobia

- Positive Kernig's sign (pain and resistance on passive knee extension with hips fully flexed)

- Non-blanching rash (Roll a glass over lesion which remains in spite of the pressure)

- Possibly seizures

- Possible focal neurological signs

- Nausea and vomiting

Meningitis 2

Investigations:

- Neurological assessment

- Lumbar puncture if safe to do so

    - May appear cloudy in bacterial meningitis

    - Clear in viral meningitis

    - Should not have blood unless infiltrated from superficial vessels in the skin.

Send for:

- Microscopy culture and sensitivity. Chromatographic evaluation may show old bleed (Xanthachronia).

- Gram stain.

- Protein estimation.

- Glucose.

- Virology.

Investigations:

- Bloods – FBC, U&Es, CRP, LFT, Coagulation screen

- Blood cultures, throat swab one for bacteria, one for virus.

- CT to rule out contraindications to LP if suspected.

Management of meningitis

Antibiotics:

- In the case of meningococcal meningitis, antibiotics should be commenced immediately.

- When treating blind:

    - Benzylpenicillin and cefotaxamine

    - Otherwise follow advice from microbiologist following return of C&S

- Consider exposure of family and friends

- Give prophylactic antibiotics

- This organism is not aerosolised and kissing contact is the level of contact that puts individuals at risk

- Isolate suspected bacterial forms

- There is no need to isolate viral meningitis in a side room.

Stroke

Presentation:

- Sudden onset or deterioration over hours or days that occurs in step to step progression.
- May have flaccid hemiplegia that becomes spastic
- May be unconsciousness
- May have dysphasia or aphasia
- Myriad of other focal and widespread neurological symptomlogy

Management:

- Rapid assessment
- Confirm diagnosis of a thrombus or bleed on CT scan
- Treatment within 3 hours of onset of symptoms
- Thrombolysis with anteplase (t-PA) for thrombus strokes

Contraindications to Thrombolysis:

- Major infarction on CT
- Recent surgery
- Active bleed from some other site
- Coagulopathy or anticoagulant – Assess on coagulation screen
- Past CNS haemorrhage

Stroke management where thrombolysis is not indicated

- NBM until swallow reflex assessed as present.

- Hydration with IVI. Try not to overly hydrate as can worsen cerebral oedema

- Mobilise and turn in bed.

- Monitor BP and do not let hypotension occur, caution with managing hypertension.

- Initially ECG monitoring, AF is common co-finding.

- Monitor oxygen saturations to prevent hypoxia, which can worsen cerebral injury.

Common complications to observe for:

- Aspirational pneumonia due to poorly guarded airway.

- Infection due to immobility UTI, chest infection.

Chapter 10 – Further reading

Chapter 10: Further Reading

Shah S	1999	Neurological assessment Nursing times 13, 49-56
De Dombel FT, ed	1993	Surgical decision making Butterworth Oxford
Brian D Rakesh R,	1999	Post operative care of the patient Student BMJ April
Fuller, G	2004	*Neurological examination made easy* Churchill Livingstone, London
Hickey, J	2002	*The Clinical Practice of Neurological and Neurosurgical nursing* Lippincott, Williams and Wilkins

Chapter 11

Nurse prescribing of drugs

In November of 2005 the Secretary of State announced an extension of nurse prescribing which came into effect in the spring of 2006.

A specifically identified group of nurses, described as an *Extended formulary nurse prescribe* will, after undertaking specialist training, be able to prescribe any licensed medicine, which now includes control drugs, such as Diamorphine for identified conditions.

The implications for nursing as a profession are far reaching, in that this new function uncouples nurses from the prescription within the context of pre decided and established problems and treatment pathways. It will rapidly bring the nurse to a position where the task of prescription is reconciled with an identified rationale that the nurse has recognised.

For the nurse this change will bring a much greater focus on the need for a skill set that has great depth and forcefully underpins the inevitable growth in professional autonomy.

The challenge for the nurse as an individual practitioner is to ensure that their practice is resoundingly robust, in that it is always underpinned by a structure and process that assures a qualitative approach. It must also always bring to the patient the best care, all within a framework of risk reduction and safest approach.

Each time a nurse uses this enhancement of prescribing with in their role, they need to do so in a way that makes clear and evident a process of examination, problem definition and rationale for action.

Chapter 11 Contents

Nurse prescribing: The approach

The nurse prescriber will need to create a record with a clear documented chronology of approach that has the following vital steps:

- Presenting problem.

- Past medical history.

- Known allergies and intolerances.

- Information from examination.

- Initial impression.

- Imperative to treat.

- Plan of exploration and tests.

- Statement of findings.

- Rationale for treatment choice.

A standard for nurse prescription

Documentation of initial contact with patient and findings and outcome. Documentation of patients consent within the patient record.

- The intended patient should be identified on the prescription by their:

    - Name and date of birth.

    - Hospital or NHS number.

    - Address, particularly for the community patient.

- Known allergies must be noted otherwise **NO KNOWN ALLEGIES** should be documented.

- The patient's weight should be recorded.

- A corresponding record of the prescribed drugs should be written in the patient's notes.

- The nurse prescriber should sign their name and print legibly their full name and professional designation.

The prescription

- The prescription should be clearly written in black ink or computer generated.

- Drug names should not be abbreviated.

- The dose should be written in clear numbers with no unnecessary decimal points, for example:

4mg and not 4.0mg

1 gram should be written as 1gm and not 1.0gm

- An amount less than a gram should be described in "mg". For example:

500mg and not 0.5gm

- Similarly quantities less than a milligram should be written in microgram.

- If it is impossible to avoid a decimal point then it should be proceeded by a zero as:

0.5 ml of solution not .5ml

- Microgram should not be abbreviated.

- Dose and frequency should be clearly stated and if the prescription chart allows, identify when each dose should be given.

- In PRN prescription the minimal dose frequency should be stated.

- Always use English and avoid Latin instructions.

An example of a prescription sheet with all the attendant information completed

SOMEWHERE HOSPITAL NHS TRUST

DRUG PRESCRIPITION AND ADMINISTRATION

WARD	WARD 17		CONSULTANT	
Unit No	1283747 P.		NURSE PRESCRIBER	Bleep No 0165
SURNAME	WHYTE		SPEACIALITY	Sug
FIRST NAME	Russel.			
DATE OF BIRTH	23\12\63			
Patients weight	75kgs.			

DRUG ALLERGIES		Nurse/Dr signature
YES(NO)NOT KNOWN	None.	Date 12/2/06
SPECIFY DRUG	N/A	~

Once only prescriptions

Date	Drug	Dose	Time	Route	Prescriber Signature	Time Given	Given By	Pharmacy
12/2/06	Cydizine	50mg	10AM	O	~	10AM	✓	

What follows next in this chapter is a resource for the clinician that will help as an easy thumb through resource. It can be used to check some of the more common prescriptions and regimes.

This chapter is intended to complement other chapters in this book, and also be used alongside recourses such as the British National Formulary (BNF), which will give extended text regarding interactions, further cautions and other pharmacological options.

Thumb through list

- Analgesics

- Drugs used in emergencies

- Prescribing intravenous fluids

- Anti-coagulation management

- Rapid sedation

- Antibiotics

- Laxatives, sleeping tablets, anti emetics

Analgesics for mild to moderate pain

Analgesics for mild to moderate pain		
Drug	**Indication**	**Dose and frequency**
Aspirin	Mild pain	300 to 900mg every 4 to 6 hours
Aspirin	Antiplatelet prophylaxis	75 to 300mg Daily 300mg one off dose in ACS
Co-codamol	Mild to moderate pain	8mg (codeine phosphate / 500mg paracetamol) 1 to 2 tablets 4 to 6 hourly. Daily maximum of 8 tablets.
Co-dydramol 10/500	Mild to moderate pain	Dihydrocodeine 10mg / 500mg paracetamol 1 to 2 tablets 4 to 6 hourly. Daily maximum of 8 tablets
Paracetamol	Mild painPyrexia	1gm 4 to 6 hourly up to maximum of 4gm daily
Dihydrocodeine tartrate	Moderate pain to severe	30 to 60mg every 4 to 6 hours: Oral IM 50mg 4 to 6 hourly.

Strong analgesic for moderate to severe pain

Strong analgesic for moderate to severe pain		
Drug	**Indication**	**Dose and frequency**
Morphine sulphate	Severe pain	Injection 10, 15, 20, 30 mg/ml
		Infusion 1mg/1ml
Diamorphine hydrochloride	Severe pain	IM 5mg every 4 hours
Diamorphine hydrochloride	AMI	IV 5mg followed by 2.5mg slowly at 1mg/minute
Diamorphine hydrochloride	Pulmonary oedema	IV 2.5 to 5mg slowly at 1mg/minute
MST (Modified release)	Severe pain	Variable dose – 10mg to 100mg BD
Pethidine	Moderate to severe pain	50 to 150mg every 4 hours: Orally for severe pain. 50 to 100mg IM for acute pain.
Buprenorphine (Temgesic)	Moderate to severe pain	Sublingually 200 to 400 micrograms every 8 hours
Sevredol (Morphine sulphate tablets)	Severe pain uncontrolled by other opiates	10 to 50mg every 4 hours
Codeine phosphate	Mild to moderate pain	30 to 60mg every 4 hours: Orally Max of 240mg in 24 hours. IM 30 to 60mg every 4 hours.

Drugs used in emergencies and acute situations

Drugs used in emergencies and acute situations		
Drug	**Indication**	**Dose and frequency**
Adrenaline	Cardiac arrest	1mg IV every 3 to 5 minutes.
Adrenaline	Anaphylaxis	500 micrograms IM once and again in 5 minutes if there is no improvement.
Atropine	Bradycardia	300 to 600 micrograms IV, then repeat as necessary.
Adenosine	SVT	6mg over 2 seconds IV, then repeated at 2 minutes, then 12mg at 4 minutes if no response.
Amiodarone	VF refractory to shocks SVTs AF Atrial flutter	300mg IV then a further 150mg IV Aim total of 1.2g over 24 hours.
Amiodarone	SVT AF Atrial flutter	**Oral dose** 200mg TDS 1/52 then 200mg BD 1/52 then 200mg daily.
Furosemide	Acute left ventricular failure	40 to 80mg IV. **Caution as may lower K+**
Furosemide	Oliguria	40mg orally in the morning to a maintenance dose of 20mg daily.
Potassium 20mmols in 0.9% normal saline.	Hypokalemia	IV infusion 0.15% 500ml over 4 hours. **Caution: May cause arrhythmias use a cardiac monitor.**

Drugs used in emergencies and acute situations		
Drug	**Indication**	**Dose and frequency**
Potassium effervescent (Sando K) - 12mmols per tablet	Hypokalemia	2 tablets every 24 hours **Monitor serum K+**
Glucose 20%	Acute insulin induced Hypoglycaemia	20% glucose in 100ml IV Repeat if necessary
Glucagon	Hypoglycaemia Hypoglycaemia where IV access is problematic	1mg IM
Chlorpheniramine	Anaphylaxis	10 to 20mg slow IV or IM
Glyceryl Trinitrate	Chest pain associated with ACS	1 to 2 500 microgram tablets 1 to 2 400 microgram S/L sprays
Oxygen	Anaphylaxis Acute severe asthma Acute coronary Syndrome Acute pulmonary oedema Bradycardia Convulsive epilepticus	60% at 10 litres via re-breath bag
Oxygen	Mild and moderate asthma	24% to 40%
Oxygen	Mild COPD	24% to 28%
Oxygen	Severe COPD	24%
Take care with CO_2 retainers as oxygen can compromise their respiratory drive.		

Drugs used in emergencies and acute situations		
Drug	**Indication**	**Dose and frequency**
Naloxone	Reversal of opiate overdose	IV 400 micrograms followed by 100 micrograms every minute until respiratory rate > 8 rpm
Flumazenil	Reversal of sedative effects of benzodiazepines such as diazepam or diazemuls	IV 200 micrograms followed by 100 micrograms every minute until respiratory rate > 8 rpm
Diazepam	Status Epilepticus	IV 10mg emulsion: Can be given rectally if no IV access
Lorazepam	Convulsion	IV 4mg over 1 to 2 minutes
Hydrocortisone	Acute asthma COPD Anaphylaxis	IV 200mgs
Prednisolone	Acute asthma COPD Suppression of allergic and inflammatory disorders	5mg orally in acute management. 10 to 20mg daily, in severe disease anything up to 60mg daily.
Caution: Steroids can cause adrenal suppression		
Salbutamol	Asthma COPD	2.5mg to 5mg in 2.5ml via nebuliser
Salbutamol	Acute severe & moderate asthma	5mg in 2.5ml
Salbutamol	Life threatening asthma	5mg in 2.5ml with Ipratropium bromide 500 micrograms
Salbutamol	Mild to moderate COPD	2.5mg to 5mg in 2.5ml via nebuliser.

Drugs used in emergencies and acute situations		
Drug	**Indication**	**Dose and frequency**
Salbutamol	Severe COPD	5mg in 2.5ml with Ipratropium bromide 500 micrograms
Salbutamol	Other reversible airway obstruction such as broncospasm associated with anaphylaxis	2.5mg to 5mg in 2.5ml via nebuliser
Salbutamol inhaler	Reversible airway obstruction	100 to 200 micrograms 1 to 2 puffs for persistent symptoms or prophylactically in exercise induced.
Salbutamol inhaler	Reversible airway obstruction	100 to 200 micrograms 1 to 2 puffs for persistent symptoms or prophylaxis in exercise induced asthma.
Salbutamol intravenous preparation	Reversible airway obstruction	As infusion 5 micrograms per minute

Intravenous fluid prescriptions

Principles:

- Maintain normal fluid balance.

- Replace additional fluid and electrolyte loss.

- Take care with special cases, such as heart failure.

Regime		
Dextrose 5% Normal saline 0.9%	2 litres 1 litre	Over 24 hours
Supplement (Monitor electrolytes)	20-30mmols Potassium	Over same 24 hours

Replace fluid loss	Consider amount and type of fluid lost Look at fluid chart Drains Febrile loss Consider insensible losses

Reconcile fluid loss records to a fluid assessment JVP Evidence of oedema (Relative to serum proteins) Basal crackles CVP Skin turgor

Heart failure	Poor tolerance to fluid overload which can result in pulmonary oedema

| Options:
Normal saline 0.9%
Haemaccel / Gelofusin | Hypovolaemia | 1 litre over 15 to 20 minutes titrated to response |

Caution with the elderly or history of ischemic heart disease as large volumes in short space of time can precipitate a further ischemic event.

| Options:
Blood – packed cells or whole.

Cross matched if available
O negative, if not.

Haemaccel / Gelofusin if blood not available.

Normal saline 0.9% | Shock and Hypovolaemia secondary to bleeding. | Infused rapidly and titrated to response. |

Anti coagulation (Low molecular weight heparin)

Anti coagulation (Low molecular weight heparin)		
Drug	**Indication**	**Dose and frequency**
Dalteparin sodium	DVT prophylaxis prior to surgery	Regime 1: 2,500 units subcutaneous 1 to 2 hours before surgery. 2,500 units once daily for 5 to 7 days
Dalteparin sodium	DVT prophylaxis prior	Regime 2: **High Risk** 2,500 units subcutaneous 1 to 2 hours before surgery. 2,500 units 8 to 12 hours later to surgery
Dalteparin sodium	DVT prophylaxis prior to surgery	Regime 3: **High Risk** 5,000 units subcutaneous the evening before surgery. 5,000 units once daily for 5 to 7 days.

Treatment of DVT & PE with Subcutaneous Dalteparin sodium low molecular weight heparin.

Weight	Dose
46 to 56kg	10,000 units
57 to 68kg	12,500 units
69 to 82kg	15,000 units
83kg and above	18,000 units

Low molecular weight heparin is more predictable in its effect than standard heparin so can be given once or twice daily without need of monitoring.

Anti coagulation with unfractionated heparin

Anti coagulation with unfractionated heparin		
Drug	Indication	Dose and frequency
Unfractionated heparin (Standard heparin)	Treatment for DVT or PE	Initial dose IV 5000iu. Continuous infusion of 15-25iu/kg/hour. Or subcutaneous heparin 15,000iu twice daily.

Assembly:

- 25,000 iu heparin to gross volume 50mls with normal saline 0.9%.

- Strength 500 iu per ml.

- Infused at between 2 and 4ml per hour, titrated to activated partial prothrombin time (APTT).

- Monitoring APTT every 10 hours.

APTT	Change rate by units per hour
5 to 7	-500
4 to 5	-300
3 to 4	-100
2.5 to 3	-50
1.5 to 2.5	0
1.2 to 1.4	+200
Less than 1.2	+400

If APTT is greater than 7, stop IV and check again in 4 hours.

Sedation and management for the rapid control of the acutely disturbed patient

- Initially explore non-pharmaceutical approaches.
- De-escalation. See chapter 9.
- If no response give:

Step 1

Droperidol 10mg IM and

Lorazepam 2mg IM or IV

Or

Step 2

Haloperidol up to 10 mgs IV **and**

Diazepam up to 10mg IV

Do not exceed 40mg Haloperidol or 40mg diazepam in 24 hours

If no response after 20 minutes:

Step 3

Give Clopixol Acuphase 100 to 150mg IM

Peaks at 24 to 36 hours, effective up to 72 hours.

May need to repeat steps 1 or 2 again

Antibiotics

Antibiotics		
Drug	**Indication**	**Dose and frequency**
Benzylpenicillin	Meningococcal disease Pneumonia Throat infections Otitis media Streptococcal endocarditis	IV infusion 2.4gm every 4 hours IM or slow IV 600mg to 1.2gm QDS 1.2gm every 4 hours
Flucloxacillin	Staphylococci	Oral: 250 to 500mg QDS IM: 250 to 500mg QDS IV: 250mg to 2gm QDS
Augmentin	Infections where amoxicillin alone is inappropriate	600mg to 1.2gm TDS IV 375mg to 650mg TDS orally
Amoxicillin	Broad spectrum AB: UTI, community acquired pneumonia	500mg TDS IV 250mg TDS orally
Ampicillin	Broad spectrum AB: UTI, community acquired pneumonia	500mg QDS IV 250mg - 1gm QDS orally
Cefuroxime	Infection due to sensitive gram positive and gram negative bacteria	Orally 250mg BD IV or IM 750mg QDS
Ceftazidime	Infection due to sensitive gram positive and gram negative bacteria	Orally 250mgs BD IV or IM 1gm TDS
Ceftriaxone	Infection due to sensitive gram positive and gram negative bacteria	IV or IM 1gm daily
Aztreonam	Gram negative infections	IV 1gm TDS

Antibiotics		
Drug	**Indication**	**Dose and frequency**
Meropenem	Gram positive & gram negative infections	IV 500mgs TDS
Tetracycline	Exacerbation chronic bronchitis Chlamydia	Orally: 250 to 500mg QDS
Doxycycline	Exacerbation chronic bronchitis Chlamydia Prostatitis Pelvic inflammatory disease	Orally: 200mg first day then 100mg daily
Oxytetracycline	Exacerbation chronic bronchitis Chlamydia	250 - 500mg QDS
Gentamicin	Broad spectrum aminoglycoside Septicaemia Meningitis CNS infections Pyelonephritis Prostatitis Pneumonia in hospital Endocarditis (With other ABs) Prophylaxis following urinary catheterisation	IV 3-5mg/kg daily
Caution with renal insufficiency. Serum gentamicin levels should be recorded twice a week, more if renal impairment.		

Antibiotics		
Drug	**Indication**	**Dose and frequency**
Amikacin	Serious gram negative infections resistant to gentamicin	IV 15mg/kg daily
Erythromycin	Alternative to penicillin in hypersensitive patients	Orally: 250 - 500mg QDS
Clarithromycin	Respiratory tract infection Soft tissue infections Ottis media	Orally 250mgs BD
Chloramphenicol	Potent broad spectrum antibiotic	Orally 50mg/kg/daily in 4 divided doses IV: 50mg/kg/daily in 4 divided doses
Caution: Risk of anaphylactoid response if rapidly infused Serum level needs assessment after 3 doses, earlier in renal impairment Rotate infusion site as damaging to vessels		
Co-trimoxazole	Acute exacerbation of chronic bronchitis Otis Toxoplasmosis	IV 960mgs BD

Laxatives, anti-emetics and sleeping tablets

Laxatives, anti-emetics and sleeping tablets		
Drug	**Indication**	**Dose and frequency**
Lactulose	Constipation (May take up to 48 hours)	15mls twice daily
Liquid paraffin	Constipation	10-30ml at night
Senokot	Constipation (8-10 hours to work)	2-4 tablets at night
Cyclizine	Nausea & vomiting	Oral or IV/IM 50mgs
Metoclopramide	Nausea & vomiting	Oral or IV/IM 10mgs
Temazepam	Insomnia	10-20mg at night
Flurazepam	Insomnia	15-30mg at night
Zopiclone	Insomnia	7.5mg at night 3.75mg for the elderly

Common abbreviations	
a.c.	Ante cibum – Before food
b.d.	Bis die – Twice daily
o.d.	Omni die – Once daily
o.m.	Omni mane – In the morning
p.c.	Post cibum – After food
p.r.n.	Pro re nata – When required
q.d.s.	Quarter die sumendus – 4 times daily
q.q.h.	Quarter quaque hora – Every 4 hours
Stat	Immediately
t.d.s.	Ter die sumendus – 3 times daily

Chapter 11 – Further reading

Chapter 11: Further Reading

Cresswell J	1999	Nurse prescribing handbook Association of nurse prescribing and community nurse UK
Department of Health	1999	Review of prescribing, supply and administration of medicines: Final report Crown three, The Stationery Office London
Josha A King T (Eds)	1996	Guy's Hospital nursing drug reference Mosby, London
O'Conner N	2006	Prescription for change RCN Magazine 21-25
Dougherty L, Lister S (Eds)	2004	The Royal Marsden Hospital Manual of Clinical Nursing Practice 6th Edition Blackwell, London
Kakkar VV, Boeckl O et al	1997	Efficacy and safety of low molecular weight heparin and standard unfractionated heparin for prophylaxis of post operative venous thrombus European multi centre trial. World journal of surgery21 (1): 2-9

Chapter 12

Operational management

Operational management, as a skills set, sits alongside the everyday skills of nurse, carer or doctor.

However, this chapter is primarily concerned with the healthcare worker who has responsibility of a more global nature, above and beyond the ward or clinical area. Typically these might include senior nurses, site managers, duty managers, practice managers, and site nurse practitioners.

Chapter 12 Contents

Managing the missing patient

In the hospital environment patients and clients who are in receipt of our care go missing, which presents a problem to the attendant professional.

Initially a risk assessment needs to be carried out, which is the consideration of risk to the patient associated with the following:

- Competence.

- Vulnerability.

- Physical ill health.

Competency is key and the most important consideration as, outside of any legal mechanism of restraint (See chapter 16), there is no mandate for restricting or containing a patient if they wish to leave the premises.

Competency checklist:

- Known confused state.

- Known mental illness that might affect their competency.

- Was the patient under the influence of alcohol, drugs or any other agent that might have compromised their competency?

- Physical illness that may affect mental function, for example worsening hypoxia.

- State of extreme emotion prior to leaving which may have undermined their competency.

Managing the missing patient: Actions

With the vulnerable patient action needs to be taken immediately as this situation constitutes an emergency.

- Close the environment down so that the missing patient cannot exit the building.

- Initiate a search close to the place the missing patient was last seen.

- Initiate a wider search site wide using security staff if available on site.

- Ensure a full description of the patient and what they were last wearing has been recorded.

- Contact the next of kin as they may well have information of value, and to ask them to call the unit if the patient arrives home.

- Review CCTV footage if available to establish if the patient left the building.

- Call extra resource for the site search if a big site.

- Contact the police if the patient has left the building.

- Document all action contemporaneously with time stamp for each action.

Dealing with complaints

It is common for operational managers to deal with complaints, and what is often presented at this stage is the opportunity for meaningful intervention close to the time the incident that prompted the complaint happened.

Many complaints, if dealt with promptly, can be resolved at that time and prevent escalation to a third party.

Approach:

- Listen to the complainant in a way that communicates respect.

- Demonstrate a willingness to help.

- Be clear about your status as this communicates that the complaint is being taken seriously and you have the power to deal with problems if necessary.

- Present yourself as being considered, fair and authoritative.

- Make clear the process of escalation beyond the initial meeting.

- Try to be objective with out compromising your colleagues.

Dealing with complaints: Actions

Listen to the complainant. Make notes if the complaint is complex and likely to be referred back to.

- Make a plan that is communicated to the complainant.

- Investigate as much as is possible immediately.

If the complaint is about a member of staff:

- Be fair with the member of staff and complainant.

- In extreme problems of high risk or malpractice, it maybe that staff need to be removed from the work environment immediately. See further in this chapter.

Possible interventions at this stage:

- Information and explanation.

- Where conflict has developed with a patient or their relatives and a member of staff, consider separation and possibly moving the patient to another ward.

If the complaint is about service provision:

- Identify the area of concern.

- Make a plan of investigation and management.

For example, for complaints about the food or cleaning, the plan of action may be to contact the manger responsible for this service.

Generic actions:

Always give the following information in a written format:

- Patient Advice and Liaison (PALS) service contact details.

- Instructions about how to make a complaint.

Documentation and communication:

- Ensure that complaint is fully documented.

- E-mail or write to the PALS department as a matter of course.

- Email or write to the area or service manager detailing complaint.

Incident reporting

The purpose of incident reporting is to enable organisations to have access to this information and help them respond to:

- Risk.

- Litigation management.

- Complaints management.

- Future service development and delivery.

Extensive study has shown that most unintentional failures are not down to one cause. They are usually imbedded within a complex interaction between a varied set of elements. These include human behaviour, technology, socio-cultural factors and organisational weaknesses.

The purpose of incident reporting in many organisations is to place clinical governance at the centre of policy and operational function.

Typically incident forms have a format that allows for:

- A record of the event being reported.

- A record of actions taken at time of event.

- Demographics of the individuals involved.

Incident forms are in triplicate with copies for:

- Risk management department.

- Area manager.

- Local manager (Remains in book).

Suspending staff

There are times when situations occur that are serious, or where an individual is compromised, that it is appropriate to remove them from the workplace. One of the mechanisms available is suspension.

Suspension is a neutral act and is intended to create a safe environment with the opportunity to gather information. This information will define the next step, which will be reinstatement to the workplace for the individual suspended, or if fault is found, the use of the disciplinary structure.

Many of the situations that prompt the action of suspension are open to interpretation. It may be an approach that considers cause in the context of illness is entirely appropriate, and in which the individual will take sick leave that can begin immediately.

Unusual behaviour and the use of drugs and alcohol all have an interpretation that could be considered pathological causation. However if one is using this approach to remove somebody from the workplace it must be come with a plan of action where a structure of assessment and management is defined in collaboration with occupational health department.

Whenever this situation occurs, it is essential to include the human resource department at the earliest opportunity, before suspension if possible. However if this occurs out of hours this may not be possible, particularly if the situation is so serious action has to happen immediately.

The situations that might prompt such an action are:

• Allegations of violence to patients or co-workers.

• Use of drugs or alcohol.

• Allegations of sexual misconduct in the workplace.

• Gross incompetence.

• Theft.

• Misappropriation of drugs within intent to use or misuse them, particularly controlled drugs.

• Any criminal act within the course of the working day.

• Unusual behaviour consistent with a sudden onset of severe psychotic mental illness.

• Severe breach of organisational policy, which impacts on the safety, risk and reputation of the organisation.

Suspending staff: The process for suspension

Assessment:

- Seek advice from HR department, if in hours.

- Seek advice from senior and peer colleagues, if available.

- Always have a witnessed environment when conducting interviews with any party involved.

- Use a neutral tone and stances when conducting the suspension.

- Document everything that is said.

- Ensure witness accounts are documented of whatever incident has prompted this suspension.

Advice to staff being suspended:

- Allow the staff member to be accompanied or supported by a colleague when taking them to a private location.

- Explain to the staff member the reason for suspension.

- Advise the staff member that suspension is a neutral act.

- Advise the staff member that until suspension is lifted they are not allowed on to the organisation's site, or allowed to contact any staff from the organisation regarding the alleged incident.

- Advise the staff member that they should seek support from their professional body and union.

- Advise the staff member to write an account of whatever incident has prompted the suspension after they have left the site.

Exclusion of difficult patients and relatives

Increasingly staff are finding that they have to deal with violence, aggression and anti-social behaviour from patients and relatives. The NHS executive has stated this is unacceptable and has a policy of zero tolerance to violence.

To make zero tolerance real, staff need to be empowered with a robust structure and approach that enables the identification of unacceptable behaviour, and allows a process of escalating action that contains this behaviour.

Unacceptable behaviour:

- Physical violence to staff.

- Physical violence to other patients or members of the public.

- Threats of violence.

- Violence to property.

- Offensive or threatening language.

- Other criminal acts such as theft or drug dealing.

The exclusion of a patient from a healthcare environment is difficult. As professionals we have a duty of care to the patient. We also have to balance carefully our actions of maintaining safety in line with the Health & Safety at Work Acts, and the duty of care implicit within our contractual agreement, and endorsed by the code of conduct of both nursing and medicine.

However the relationship with the relatives of the patient is an informal one and not legally subject to the same duty of care. This can make their management in the instance of anti social behaviour different, in that they can be asked to leave and reasonably kept away from the organisational site.

The process – assessment and identification of behaviour

Actions should be an ascending ladder of options that can be allocated according to the level of behaviour displayed. The intention is to change the behaviour before reaching the extreme of complete exclusion.

Option one – A letter

A letter, by hand or by post, to the individual stating the displayed behaviour is unacceptable and further action could be taken. This should also be documented in the relative's medical notes.

Option two – Relocation of treatment

This is applied where an individual has an on-going relationship with the healthcare environment but has behaved in a way that is unacceptable and if not in need of on-going care would be excluded.

To enable this approach the organisation has to enter in to a reciprocal agreement with another care provider who is prepared to exchange patients of this type.

This should also be documented in the relative's medical notes.

Option three – Exclusion

When this happens, the patient is informed that they will no longer be treated. If they are in need of care they should approach another organisation.

Fire Management

As the senior manager with responsibilities for operational management, a key responsibility is a competent response to fire.

The purpose of the senior manager is to:

- Ensure prompt and robust process of communication.
- Good management in liaison with fire officer in command.

Actions:

- On receipt of fire call ensure that the Fire Service has been called.
- If a large scale fire, set up a control centre distant from the fire so the management of response is not compromised by the fire itself
- Wear the fire marshal vest
- Be the point of contact for services
- Ensure radio communication available
- Appoint an evacuee marshal
- Identify a safe point for evacuation
- Send extra staff to help with the evacuation without compromising the safety of staff
- Keep records of individuals evacuated.

See chapter 16 for more information on fire response.

Chapter 13

Managing a major incident

A major incident is when an extraordinarily large number of casualties have been caused by an event that may overwhelm the hospital and emergency services and therefore needs special provision.

The following chapter will deal with essential considerations for the operational manager and senior clinician when planning to receive mass casualties.

Chapter 13 Contents

Declaration of the major incident

A major incident is declared by the ambulance service at the scene and is communicated by the hotline directly to the nearest casualty.

A major incident is:

Any emergency, including known or suspected acts of terrorism, that requires implementation of special arrangements by one or all of the emergency services and will generally include the involvement, either directly or indirectly, of large numbers of people.

For example:

- The rescue and transportation of a large number of casualties.

- The mobilisation and organisation of the emergency services and support services, for example a local authority, to cater for the threat of death, serious injury or homelessness to a large number of people.

- The large scale damage to the environment or disruption to the community.

The first stage is the declaration. A formal declaration of a major incident is an important step as it serves to change the mindset of people involved to emphasise the need for strategic coordination. Secondly it triggers specific responses by individual agencies.

Once the major incident has been declared the hospital will respond by putting into action a well-rehearsed action plan to enable the hospital quickly to respond to an influx of many causalities.

Actions:

Major incident cascade bleep.

This automated series of bleeps that call in a pre-identified group of key professionals.

Command function

Formulation of the command post and the major incident controller takes up position.

The command post has three areas of key function:

- Communication.

- Deployment of resource.

- Coordination of logistics.

The communication function has the following priorities:

Action

- Ensure all wards and departments aware.

- Clear beds on receiving wards.

- Clear Accident and Emergency.

- Clear theatres and cancel any surgery planned for the day.

- Direct incoming staff to needed areas.

- Ensure extra key equipment is deployed to receiving and key areas.

- Cancel elective admissions.

Instruct communication department to set up the communication centre which will deal with:

- Anxious relatives' enquiries.

- Press enquiries.

- Receiving telephone calls from staff calling in to help.

The command function is available for information and updates from external sources:

- Fire brigade.

- Ambulance.

Also, in the instance of a developing issue such as a terrorist attack, the command centre should allocate an individual to follow news reports from the scenes and scan the internet for updates.

Instruct logistic response

- Make the site secure by deploying security staff to lock down the site.

- Instruct catering to plan for extra capacity of staff and patients.

- Clear accommodation.

- Make available extra equipment such as dressings and CSSD, for example.

Major incident: Special considerations

- Infection risk such as biological terrorism.

- Chemical risk from the same source.

If either of the above are an issue, then the logistical response will need extra resources in terms of setting up a decontamination area in the instance of chemical attack and extra barrier provision if biological hazard.

Command centre further responsibilities:

- Continually risk-assess the hospital site, particularly in the instances of terrorism.

- Consider safety of hospital site relative to workload.

- Ensure liaison with other hospitals and logistic provision for, if and when the hospital site becomes overwhelmed.

- Record all activity.

- Ensure every patient has an identity tag.

- Ensure every deceased patient has an identity tag, or efforts are made to identify them.

- Records of all patients should be made contemporaneously and communicated to both command centre and communications.

Staff may have to be kept from leaving the site, if they are contaminated.

Chapter 13 – Further reading

Chapter 13: Further Reading

Health & Safety executive	2005	Major incident response and investigation and major incident policy and procedure review Health & Safety executive publications London
Department of Health	2006	Emergency planning DOH HMSLO London
London emergency services liaison panel	2004	Major incident procedure manual
Mayoral office	2005	Mayoral statement www.london gov.uk/mayor/mayorstatement
British red cross	2005	Information sheet: London bombing British red cross, Moorfields London
Miles S	1991	Major incidents British Medical Journal (301) 923

Chapter 14

Bed management and the 4-hour Accident and Emergency target

Bed management is often considered an obvious function and a role that has a limited range of possible options to achieve the desired outcome. However, when this function comes into your remit it becomes clear that bed management is a complex and intricate process of constant juggling and manoeuvring, often just to stay in the same place.

Good bed management is fundamental to the successful management of the hospital. Without it, other functions of the hospital environment are progressively and detrimentally affected.

The need for active management of the beds has come about as occupancy has increased and often the demand outstrips the supply. Only with the diligent and active management of beds can this unworkable conundrum be resolved.

The role of bed manager came into being some twenty years ago at St. Thomas' Hospital and has been propagated as an example of best practice throughout the NHS. The original project lead, Bill Addison, is still fulfilling this role today.

In many environments the bed management role has become part of another role, such as the hospital co-ordinator, or the site nurse practitioner. However, whoever provides this function can benefit from the hints and tips to follow in this chapter.

Chapter 14 Contents

Bed Management

Bed management is a fundamental skill in all roles involving any senior bed management responsibility.

The purpose of bed management is easy enough and it involves placing patients into an appropriate bed from an admission source, typically Accident and Emergency, hospital clinics or from a GP referral. The problems start when the number of available beds is insufficient for the number of patients needing admission.

A further consideration is the government targets of all patients being seen in the Accident and Emergency department and either admitted or discharged within 4 hours.

What follows are some tips and pointers on how to manage beds with these two competing pressures.

Management of discharge

Ensure junior staff are aware of likely discharges and put in place all necessary arrangements ahead of time:

- Let nurses lead the discharge process, identifying likely or aimed for discharge dates as early as possible in the patient's care.

- Create a culture of discharge rounds happening at least the evening before discharge.

- Book transport the day before discharge.

- Ensure prescriptions for medicines to be taken home are written and dispensed the day before discharge.

- Ensure social services, home care provision is in place the day before discharge.

- Ensure relatives are on-board early, especially if they have a role in providing transport home or home care.

Ensure all beds are used

In many hospitals, beds remain empty but are recorded as full. The reason for this is often about departmental or ward level behaviour prioritising local imperatives over hospital wide considerations.

This can be argued as reasonable on the basis of having a predictable capacity for planning of elective workload and also making beds available for other specialities and can be problematic in terms of the quality of care for the patient out of area.

These beds are held or blocked for patients who are elsewhere, for example:

- Intensive Care Unit (ICU): It maybe that the patient's return is imminent or they may be in ICU for an extended period of time

- High Dependence Unit (HDU): The same as above applies

- In theatre: Again the patient may well be returning directly to the ward or in fact they may be moving through a planned period in the recovery department which maybe in excess of a day.

- Weekend leave. The patient may be away for an extended period.

- To Come In: The expected date of admission may be some time away.

- Broken bed

- Issues of infection control: In many environments where a side room is not available or the patient's severity of illness is considered too great a risk to have in a side room, the patient may be isolated in a more open area which will necessitate the blocking of beds adjacent to the patient.

All these issues have to be explored in detail for the possibility of extra unseen capacity.

An example of how this capacity may be used is in the instances of a weekend leave of a two day period. This may allow a short two day admission and episode of care within that same bed space which is not disrupted to either patient but maximise the use of that bed resource.

Finding and using beds of this status can cause problems for the nurse practitioner and will often be contentious. You will have to weigh up the immediate short-term advantage over the political fall out. We all have an investment in getting the job done but also and possibly equally, we need to invest in the continued cordial relations with our colleagues.

Delayed Discharges

There are always a number of patients who are in a hospital bed beyond their medical need, invariably they are elderly with complex needs which involve social services input and they are waiting for placement in a care setting.

Movement of these patients can make a significant difference to the overall function of the hospital particularly if there are a number of them.

In a day-to-day function it may be difficult to move this on, but strategically there are options available. The first being to ensure the social services department are aware of the patient and have awarded a high priority in their records. This will involve daily communication from the discharge manager, if the role exists within the hospital in which you work.

Have a process of escalation where key milestones are scheduled and, if missed or do not produce the desired effect, have a higher level of escalation.

A key part of the process is banding where the level of needed care is decided, this is often delayed within the hospital environment as various clinicians involved do not consider this process a priority.

Having this meeting promptly, and as soon as it is decided that the patient no longer has physical needs, will mean that any delays beyond this period becomes the responsibility of social services.

Social services often meet on a monthly or bi-monthly schedule. It is important to ensure banding happens ahead of these meetings so as to avoid a delay waiting for a banded patient waiting for the next sitting of the social services panel.

The whole process has a dependency on many different professions across the acute hospital and community environment, which can lead to long delays. A way to push this forward is to actively manage the process ensuring all parties see each patient referral as high priority.

Managing the movement of patients into the hospital

In times of acute need it may be appropriate to look at the elective admission list to see if there is an opportunity to maximise use of all bed resources by admitting pre-operative patients to a hotel environment rather than an acute bed.

Patients pre-operatively may be well and have no care needs until they are in the post-operative period.

Some hospitals will cancel elective admissions in the instance of a crisis. If you are in this position remember to have a process of decision-making that looks at the following:

- Clinical need. Patients with cancer and immediate life threatening conditions should never be cancelled.

- Prioritise patients that have previously been cancelled.

- How long has the patient been waiting? This cancellation may put the patient outside the expectable and stipulated waiting period for this procedure.

Remember cancelling a patient is very disruptive and stressful for them. Consider cancellation as a very last resort.

Emergency Bed Service (EBS)

There are opportunities to manage patient admission rate, which is an escalating process of containment relative to the increasing inability of the hospital to cope with the admission volumes.

The EBS has a role of coordinating the emergency and urgent admission traffic. They have the following options at their disposal:

Own District Only (ODO) is a status where the EBS will change the open status of the hospital to a lesser level where the hospital will not accept patients from outside the hospital district when referred from GPs.

EBS will want to know:

• What admission activity you have had through Accident and Emergency in the last 24 hours?

• How many patients are currently waiting in Accident and Emergency?

• What elective admissions have been placed on hold or in a bed?

Once EBS has accepted the request to change the status of the hospital you will need to contact the registrars of the admitting teams and tell them:

- Change of status.

- What areas are within district.

- Refer any GP requests to EBS.

Medical Referral Only (MRO) is a status greater than ODO, where patients even from the hospitals district are referred back to EBS for placement elsewhere. This is potentially problematic because of knock on events as:

- Patients may not be accessible to relatives visiting if placed far away.

- Increased complaints.

- Retrieval back may be difficult, adding pressure on another day in the future.

Ambulance divert is a more extreme manoeuvre which is brought into play when there is an extreme event such as a fire in the Accident and Emergency department, or the hospital is the site of a massive disruptive event.

An ambulance divert involves the CEO calling their equivalent in another hospital and asking them to take ambulance admissions for a period of time.

Discharge rounds

In the instance of an acute bed crisis, a useful manoeuvre is to instigate a discharge round where a senior clinician, usually at consultant level, is instructed to carry out a ward round identifying patients that can be discharged immediately, rather than at some point in the future. There are usually a number of patients in hospital who could be discharged but are awaiting non-clinical intervention.

This approach carries risk as patients may be discharged without a structured care package or some other significant elements are not in place. As always, risk needs to be reduced to a minimum, if the risk remains too great then the discharge cannot go ahead.

Opening beds

Many hospitals will consider opening extra beds in a crisis; these may consist of an extra bed on each ward or an extra area being used as a new clinical area.

This approach to managing a crisis can be a useful short term intervention but it carries many problems in that extra beds need extra staff and areas not designed for housing patients will be missing key equipment and infrastructure.

The Accident and Emergency 4-hour wait

This government initiative has had a dramatic affect on the way hospitals function. Since that time, Accident and Emergency departments have had to spend an increasing amount of time policing their own practice and enforcing patient movement from the department within the 4-hour period.

In many hospitals the response to this new imperative is to create a role with the specific responsibilities to enable rapid management of the patient to ensure compliance with the target time. This role comes from either within the Accident and Emergency department or outside. Either way, it is the responsibility of anyone with global site responsibility.

Tips for achieving the 4-hour target:

- Pay close attention to the time line and ensure a plan of action exists early on in the 4-hour period.

- Ensure key tasks are identified, such as referral to accepting team.

- Keep an eye open to potential problems such as failure of the CT scanner or the pneumatic blood sample delivery system, or a particular team of doctors who are slow to respond to referral.

- Have a ward designated for short term stays, such head injuries secondary to alcohol consumption. This ward area can have two functions. The first is to take patients that will need a short term admission and the second is to take patients who are waiting for a diagnostic outcome that may fall outside the 4-hour period

- This designated ward area should run with spare capacity if possible and be physically close to the Accident and Emergency department.

Many hospitals have beds within a hotel environment on hospital grounds that can accommodate relatives of sick patients, in addition to well patients who have a delay in their discharge for some reason.

Chapter 14 – Further reading

Chapter 14: Further Reading		
Dash K et al	1996	Discharge planning for the elderly. a guide for nurse Springer New York
Department of health	2004	Faster access :Bed management demand and discharge predictors HSMLO London
Department of health	2004	Toolkit – wait for a bed: Bed management further guidance HSMLO London
Audit commission	2003	Bed management Audit Commission Publications Yorkshire
Clare O'Brian	2003	Bed management policy St Peters Ashford www.ashfordstpeters.nhs.co.uk
Department of health	2002	Bed occupancy Department of Health Hospital activity web site
Brimlow A	2004	Overcrowded hospitals breed MRSA: Overcrowded hospitals are providing a breeding ground for the super bug MRSA, say infection experts BBC Publications

Chapter 15

The Hospital at Night (HAN)

The Hospital at Night project is a fundamental and unprecedented new approach to the management of the hospital, and particularly the management of relations between the various professions, particularly doctors and nurses.

The new working practices that this project enforces represent a source of development for all the professional groups and consequently a source of stress and possible conflict as new roles are defined and consolidated.

For the nurse, the main concern is the expectation of leadership to their medical colleagues in the clinical and operational environment, a group who have traditionally remained outside of a cohesive management structure.

Doctors have always validated their position by reference to their exclusive body of knowledge. The nurse also challenges this relationship across the spectrum, extending and expanding their skill base into areas that were previously the preserve of the doctor alone.

The HAN project potentially positions the nurse and the nurse practitioner into two particularly difficult situations. Firstly managing a group of doctors who are reluctant to take their lead and secondly to be seen as a clinical lead in areas that are new practice to them, which is enthusiastically drawn on by the junior doctors.

These difficult and new situations can be challenging for the nurse as they are often in the minority amongst a group of doctors.

Similarly, the doctor is faced with problems of role identity and the exercise of accountability. They are forced into a situation where they have to accept the judgement and clinical input of a professional who has varying clinical training and ability.

The doctor, like all professions, is defined by the history and sociology of their particular profession. Consequently they will have an expectation of taking the lead and find it hard to adjust to these changing circumstances.

Chapter 15 Contents

Hospital at Night

The Hospital at Night project began in various pilot sites around the country in April 2003, with aim of enabling the European Working Time Directive (EWTD) and reducing the hours worked by junior doctors.

- Medical cover provided in hospitals during the out-of-hours period has been changed.

- Medical cover requirements are no longer defined by professional demarcation and grade. Cover is now based on the competence of staff in attendance.

- The project aims to enable and possibly enhance care for patients given the changes in permitted working hours of doctors in training.

- The HAN project offers a method of preserving, and even enhancing, doctors' training by reduced hours available.

- The HAN model consists of a multidisciplinary night team, which has the competences to cover a wide range of interventions. It also has the capacity to call in senior and specialist expertise when necessary.

- This model contrasts the traditional model of junior doctors working in isolation.

The project advocates

Managed multi-speciality handovers.

Other team members taking on the role and tasks formerly associated with the doctor. Typically the nurse in the practitioner role and at the bedside.

Relocating a significant portion of the non-urgent work from the night to the evening.

This initiative also advocates reducing the unnecessary duplication of work by better coordination and reducing the multiple clerking and reviews.

When managing the HAN project

• Senior level sponsorship comes from the consultants and the chief executive.

• The executive and the consultants should make un-ambivalent statements of support for this project with a mechanism of access and action when there are problems.

Structured cross medical speciality arrangements

• The junior doctors need to be clear about what areas they have responsibility for outside of their specialty and feel confident about support when working in an area they might find threatening.

Enhanced and expanded practice skills

Since the Scope of Practice initiative in 1992, there have been many nurses working in expanded and extended practice roles. Nurses have taken on skills and tasks usually associated with their medical colleagues. With this initiative there is a greater expectation on competence, when compared to previous models of skills and tasks being delineated according to role and discipline.

The implications for this new way of working are that in many situations the junior doctor may well look for guidance from the nurse with enhanced skills. This represents a fundamental change.

Ensure your nursing staff have access to good training in expanded skills that is from their own profession.

Have a process in place that demonstrates nursing leadership in practice – the project lead should be in practice and be able to demonstrate leadership skills within the clinical environment.

Operational management responsibilities night nurse practitioner (NNP) in charge

- The role of the NNP within the HAN team is to lead the team, as the NNP has a site wide hospital perspective.

- Allocation of staff particularly doctors.

- Responsiveness to incomplete or imperfect situations that inevitably crop up, such as problems of staffing within the doctors.

- Specific training in skills of chairing the hospital at night multi-disciplinary meeting.

Chairing the HAN meeting can be difficult if:

- The NNP is inexperienced in chairing meetings.

- The NNP may feel uncomfortable directing doctors.

- The NNP may also feel vulnerable if they are the only nurse at the meeting.

- Doctors may feel uncomfortable in that they are expected to hand over clinical details of patient assessment and management to a large group of their peers, who may consider the meeting an opportunity for critique and education.

- To manage the meeting there needs to be rules.

- The NNP may feel unclear about their formal and cultural authorisation to direct and allocate junior medical staff.

Managing the HAN team

A big strength of the HAN process is that somebody with an over-arching view and responsibility for the hospital is in charge. This means problems of medical staffing or disparity of workload can be addressed by moving doctors from an area of light workload to an area that is busier or less well staffed.

While this is sensible and in accord with the HAN strategy, it can be difficult to execute.

Junior doctors can feel uncomfortable about working out of area, particularly if they feel they are diluting the care that they are providing to their own patient group. Possibly more problematic is working in areas they feel unskilled in.

A way of offsetting this is to ensure allocated areas are of a commensurate specialism; a surgery doctor should be allocated to another surgical area for example. These problems may well be resolved when the junior doctors are no longer allocated to consultant teams.

When there is resistance to re-deployment, the NNP must feel supported when they act in this potentially contentious situation. Support must be evident and clear to the whole team, which enables the junior doctor if they feel the need to explain themselves to their consultant saying that it was not their decision but they were left with no choice.

Chairing the HAN meeting

- The chairperson has a hospital wide remit, invariably it is the NNP.

- The chairperson calls the meeting to order and it starts on time.

- Ground rules are known and stated at the beginning of each meeting.

Ground rules

Each member of the team to talk in turn.

Each team member should feel comfortable and any comments made by other members of the team should be constructive.

No person should dominate the meeting.

The order should be known and followed.

Everybody that should be at the meeting should attend. Each professional group should police this.

Everybody at the meeting introduces themselves by name and role.

The purpose of the meeting is to hand over pertinent information and not to get distracted by, for example, an interesting case.

There should not be any side meetings of information staff feel too trivial to give to the whole group.

This meeting is an opportunity to build a rapport and should include joint teaching. Of particular value are discussions on areas of joint practice where differing disciplines have very different roles such as the control and restraint of the violent patient.

There are times when team members fail to attend, siting workload or having little to hand over. This should be actively discouraged as they are avoiding the peer pressure effect of scrutiny about patient management or work unreasonably left undone.

* The role described here of NNP may have different names in different hospitals, such as Clinical Site Manager. This member of the team provides essentially the same role in the context of the HAN project.

Differing cultures of different members of the HAN team

The two professional groups that make up the HAN team are doctors and nurses. These groups have traditional ways of working and stylised regard for one which can have a dramatic impact on working relations.

An awareness of these cultural and social differences can greatly enable a proactive model of conflict avoidance and rapport building.

Professional cultures and conflict

These cultural characteristics exist historically and there are many examples of collaboration and new approaches by both professions that run counter to this analysis. Nevertheless, it may help to give a character of the historical position of both groups, which can shed light onto possible areas of conflict and more importantly how to resolve conflict when it arises.

Professional characteristics of doctors and nurses

Nursing	Medicine
Allegiance to organisation first	Allegiance to profession first
Centrally managed	Managed local to Doctor
Uniformity of rules and conventions	Internalised rules/values
Legal and rational bases for decision making	Scientific rationale decision making
Equally scientific and intuitive	Historically intolerant of other rationale for action
Measured competence (Certificated skill)	See one, do one, teach one (Historically)
Structure Dependent	Independent
Historically low autonomy	Pride in autonomy
Team approach	Competitive and individualistic approach
Female (Historically)	Male (historically)

Examples of conflict issues in the HAN project

Doctor is reluctant to give clinical handover to the whole team.

Handover given outside of HAN meeting.

Tasks saved and given to the only NNP.

Doctors going to bed during the course of a rostered shift of work.

Doctors not trusting nurse colleague's judgement.

Nurses not taking on decisions.

Intolerance of the limitations of nurses.

Lack of understanding about the nature of rules that govern nursing.

Both sides reluctant to take on stand alone fiddly tasks.

The day staff leaving tasks unnecessarily for the HAN teams.

Examples of conflict issues in the HAN project

Nurses falling into "Matronly" behaviour and being very prescriptive in their management style.

Nurses making decisions in anticipation of the doctor and then not having to account for those decisions.

The process of referral being dependent on a worsening condition of the patient that causes frustration to both parties.

Resolving conflict

Fundamental to building the HAN team

- Communication.

- Respect.

- Parity.

At the HAN meeting

- Make clear statement about what is expected of each team member at a very detailed level.

- Which patients should be seen and in what time frame.

- What is the trigger for referral?

- What workload should trigger a call for help?

- What extra duties may be asked of each staff member in extremis.

- What routine tasks the doctor should undertake?

- What routine tasks should be undertaken by the NNP?

Resolving conflict

What are the limits of each role?

For example a house officer in their first job should not take direct medical referrals.

It is unlikely the NNP can prescribe the same range of drugs a doctor can.

Have clear collective goals for the team.

Be clear about the responsibility of individuals to fulfil their obligations.

Explain new roles, skills and limitations – What the NNP can do and what they cannot.

Have a stable and consistent approach to each shift.

Establish a rapport.

Where possible both sides should take opportunities to teach one another.

Plan joint training sessions.

For the nurse, learn the language of the doctor but use only up to the extent of your knowledge

Show empathy by anticipating issues of workload and proactively assign staff to areas of need. For example a dermatology doctor to help the over worked medical doctor or vice versa.

Start young: Many of the newly qualified doctors state they find the HAN structure very supportive as they need and cherish the direction and support provided by senior nurses and doctors that are working alongside them.

Chapter 15 – Further reading

Chapter 15: Further Reading		
Modernisation agency	2004	Findings and recommendations from the hospital at night project: Implementation resource pack Modernisation agency London
Academy of medical royal colleges	2003	The development of an out of hours medical team Academy of medical royal colleges London
BMA Junior doctors committees	2003	Safe handover: Safe patients: Guidance on clinical handover for clinicians and managers British medical association Junior doctors committee

Chapter 16

Violence and aggression management

Violence and aggression is an increasing part of the life of the carer, whether in the hospital setting, the community or any other therapeutic environment.

The increasing incidence and severity of violence (Department of Health 2003) is putting a greater emphasis on the healthcare professional to add management of violence and aggression to their portfolio of skills. This is in order to maintain their own safety and to maintain a safe environment in which care objectives can be met.

To manage violence and aggression effectively, the healthcare professional will need to develop an extended skill set that not only enables them in the specific instance of violence, but also fundamentally changes the individual's orientation and approach.

To be effective, one has to consider the possibility of violence in all situations and plan pre-emptively.

The best outcome is that violence is avoided and aggression proactively managed.

In this chapter, the skills described will facilitate the healthcare professional with physical skills underpinned by a moral and legal frame for action planning in this volatile and difficult situation.

Chapter 16 Contents

Violence and aggression management strategies

Communication has three fundamental elements

- Verbal.

- Body language.

- Use of space.

Be aware of all three elements as a guide to how a situation may be changing.

Non para-verbal signs:

- Tone.

- Volume.

- Speed of delivery.

Signs of escalation:

- Aggressive tone.

- Increased volume.

- Increased speed of delivery.

However, there are times when an aggressor will use a flat, slow considered monotone, which can erupt seemingly without warning.

Verbal Escalation

- Screaming.

- Swearing.

- High energy.

- Dehumanisation: possible using language of sexism and racism.

- Loss of rationalisation.

- Verbal and non-verbally threatening staff.

- Taking personal space: Remember this is a changing space relative to how excitable and aggressive the individual is.

- Refusal or non-compliance.

- Questioning proceeding to challenging.

- Unable to take direction.

Body Posture: Signs of escalation

- Face to face posture.

- Moving towards individual with whom conflict is developing.

- In an aggressive situation, the need for an increase in safe space between individuals must be observed. The aggressor can interpret infringement of space as counter aggressive stance which can in turn be the flash point where aggression becomes violence.

- Chin is often lifted up.

- Hands may be concealed.

- Hands may be clenched into a fist and held to the side but slightly forward as though to indicate the readiness for physical conflict.

- Eye contact maybe staring with little or no blinking.

Strategy for management

- Initially make an assessment.

- How urgent is this situation?

- What are the risks?

- Who is at risk?

- Are there factors feeding the escalation?

- Do I need greater resource before acting?

Approaches

- Position yourself so that the exit is behind you and unobstructed

- Seek help – use a phone, emergency buzzer or consider leaving immediately. Individual intervention involves a higher risk.

- Observe the individual's personal space if the situation allows.

- In an escalating situation the aggressor's need for personal space will increase.

- Hands off – do not touch the individual even in a supportive fashion as, in this volatile state, this can be misinterpreted as an attack and pre-empt the flash point of violence.

Interventions

Consider the goal of the intervention:

- The goal should be hierarchical.

- Rapid risk assessment.

- Make the situation safe for all parties.

- Establish a rapport.

- De-escalate.

Ideally these goals can be achieved together. However, you may have to act quickly to prevent loss of life or the threat of extreme harm. In this case safety takes priority over all other matters.

If possible remove any audience, which can be a catalyst to a situation.

Allow emotional expression.

Convey an understanding emotional response when building a rapport.

Give non-threatening directives.

Enforce any limits you set.

What to do, and what not to do

Do	Do not
Position yourself safely	Rush in
Remain calm	Over react
Isolate the situation	Get in a power struggle
Enforce limits	Make false promises
Listen	Fake attention
Be aware of the non-Verbal	Be threatening
Be consistent	Use jargon, it can confuse and frustrate

Empathic listening skills

- This is an active process.

- Non-judgemental.

- Undivided attention.

- Listen with a focus on real feelings, theirs and yours.

- Allow silence for reflection.

- Use restatement to clarify message.

Use a supportive stance

- Side by side.

- Hands visible but not raised.

- This position is non-threatening or challenging.

- Communicate respect without deference.

- Honour personal space.

- Not threatening.

- By standing side on, legs apart the healthcare worker is more able to move away quickly.

- Contributes to staff members personal safety.

Precipitating factors

In planning the management of aggression and possible violence, a feeling for what might precipitate an aggressive event can be useful in proactively management.

- Loss of personal power.

- Need to maintain self-esteem.

- Fear – not knowing what is happening.

- Failure – not being able to complete a task.

- Attention seeking behaviour.

- Displaced anger.

- Severe upset related to receiving bad news such as a bereavement.

- Psychological/physiological causes.

- Drugs.

- Hypoglycaemia.

- Pain.

- Insomnia.

- Psychological disorders.

- Alcohol or substance withdrawal.

Insights as a Functional Aid

- Always plan to pre-empt the crisis that is violence and aggression.

- Depersonalise crisis: we are seldom the cause of the crisis.

- Rational detachment: to be detached from the crisis allows you to offer a therapeutic rapport building solution.

- Stay in control of own response: When feelings are running high it is easy to become emotionally involved.

- Maintain a professional attitude: Control the situation with out overreacting

- Following the management of a violent or aggressive situation, ensure that a managed debrief happens as close to the conclusion of the event as possible. This may help with closure and reflective learning.

- Beyond clinical supervision, staff should have positive outlets for negative energy absorbed from aggressive situations.

Managing yourself in an escalating situation

- Proactively manage a situation, if you know someone to be violent plan your approach.

- Where violence is part of the patient's known condition, a therapeutic management plan should be in place.

- Never attempt to manage an escalating situation alone.

- Remove yourself from a dangerous situation as soon as you feel it is getting out of control.

- Position yourself with a door behind you.

- Allow consideration where you exit.

- Summon help at the first opportunity.

- Position yourself side on, offering a lesser target in the instance of attack.

- This is also a supportive and less confrontational stance.

- Always be conscious of your client's non-verbal signs.

Block and release techniques

The block and release techniques are designed for situations where the professional is under attack. The purpose of these techniques is to enable the healthcare worker to move away quickly from a situation in order to prevent further injury from attack.

From a position of greater safety the healthcare worker can assess help with the intention of regaining control.

The following techniques are designed to allow:

- Protection from an attacking aggressor.

- Quick release when being held.

- Rapid exit of the professional from an untenable situation.

The success of these techniques depends on the use of:

- Preparation: Awareness of the para-verbal signs of agitation and potential aggression.

- Surprise: The ability to act inconsistently with the expectation of the aggressor.

- Momentum and leverage: Use of maximum strength at the point of greatest weakness.

Single hand wrist hold release

It is not uncommon for an aggressor to attempt to hold the healthcare worker by the wrist.

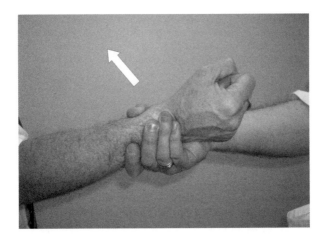

Moving quickly pull the hand up and away from the hold.

Aim your efforts at the weakest point of the hold, which is between forefinger and thumb of the aggressor.

Whilst moving your hand up, position your body to the side, with a wide gate as though making to run.

This will allow extra effort to be applied to the pulling away action.

Move your face away from your own hand which, when suddenly released, can hit your own face.

This will also allow you to move away quickly once released.

Double hand wrist hold release

It is also possible that an aggressor may use two hands to consolidate the wrist hold.

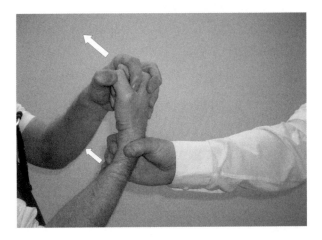

This movement also relies on applying pressure to the weak point of the grip. To add to the momentum of the move by employing the second hand extra leverage is also added.

Using two hands in this fashion the released healthcare worker will present a shoulder to the aggressor that will be moving with some force. This can catch the aggressor off guard and provide some extra time for escape.

Hair hold with one hand

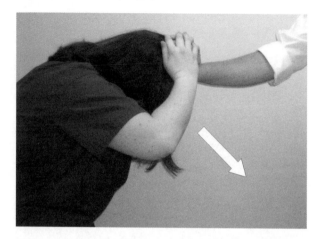

This move requires the immobilisation of the aggressors hold by clasping the aggressors hand in both hands and applying pressure down. This manoeuvre also has the effect of reducing the pain and minimising further injury.

When the hair is secured, move towards the aggressor attempting to simultaneously weaken the grip and push the aggressor off balance.

If this manoeuvre is attempted half-heartedly the aggressor can respond by tightening the grip and be kicking.

Hair hold with two hands

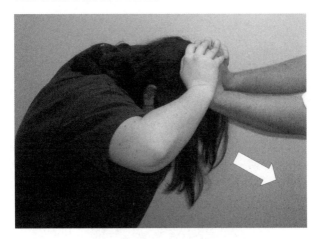

This move repeats the same element described before. However, with two hands the aggressor has a weaker grip but may well be holding the hair in an attempt to hold the professional down in order to kick the face. **Speed therefore is very important**.

Both manoeuvres will benefit from a loud shout, which will surprise the aggressor and alert colleagues in the near vicinity.

This move also requires the immobilisation of the aggressors hold by clasping the aggressors hand in both hands and applying pressure down.

Front strangle hold release

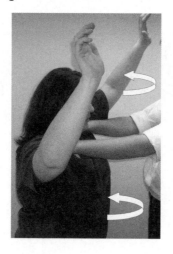

Lift both arms into the air.

Shout in order to surprise the aggressor.

Twist away from the aggressor applying pressure to the weak points of the grip.

Then move away quickly.

Do not attempt to put your arms inside the grip of the aggressor, if you successfully disengage you will be brought face to face rather than to a position of moving away.

Strangle hold from behind

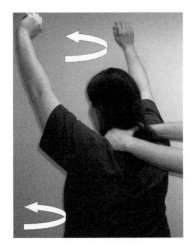

Arms up.

Shout loudly.

Step back to weaken the hold.

Then turn and twist as with the previous hold.

Then move away quickly.

Release from bite

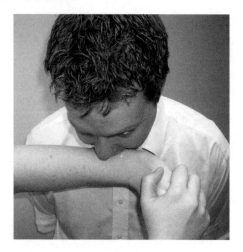

The bite is often in the arm or wrist as the professional will invariably use arms in defence, which becomes the first point of contact with the aggressor.

When bitten in this fashion, lean into the bite.

Vibrate into the aggressor's mouth which will induce a parasympathetic response causing the mouth to open.

Move away from the aggressor.

Kick avoidance

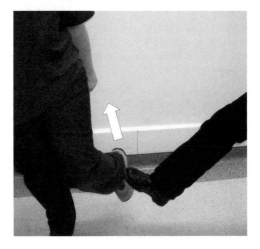

A natural response to an attack is to shield oneself. In the instance of a kick, the shield used is usually the leg.

Stand side on. Lift the leg so the aggressor makes contact with the side of the shoe, deflecting the blow and protecting those vulnerable areas of groin and abdomen.

Move away from the aggressor.

Legal mechanisms for restraint

In healthcare it is becoming increasingly common to encounter situations where restraint is used. As a professional, whether a doctor, nurse or healthcare assistant we need to be assured that what we are doing is legally defensible and reasonable.

In the following section, information will be given about the possible mechanisms at the professional's disposal but with recognition of the ambiguities that exist in the current law and the overriding principle that should always be applied, that of conscious accountability in action.

Making the decision to restrain

The decision to restrain a patient or client is a decision to restrict their movement. It is not only a decision to physically hold a person against their will, and does not necessarily involve physical contact.

The legal considerations are the same and a professional in this situation must have a structure or framework for their decision-making.

Possible rationale for holding somebody against their will:

- Irrational and violent behaviour that might result in self harm.

- Irrational and violent behaviour that might result in someone else's harm.

- Incompetence where the individual is at risk due to, for example, a confused state.

- Incompetence due cognitive impairment where there is an identified risk.

- Where someone is subject to a court order such as the 1984 Public Health Act.

- A child who has been identified at risk and separated from a responsible adult.

- Following, or during, a criminal act such as theft or violent assault.

Legal mechanisms of restraint

- Mental Health Act 1983

- Public Health Act 1984

- Common law

- Power of arrest (Public Order Act 1967)

The Mental Health Act 1983

Section	Period	Purpose	Application
Section 2	Up to 28days	Assessment	Two doctors where one has previous experience of the patient
Section 3	6 months initially	Treatment	Two doctors where one has previous experience of the patient and the other approved
Section 4	Emergency for up to 72hours		One medical recommendation in the emergency situation
Section 5(2)	Emergency for up to 72hours	Assessment	Doctor SHO or above for patients currently voluntary patients in hospital
Section 5(4)	Emergency for up to 6 hours	Assessment	Trained mental health nurse for voluntary patients currently in hospital
Section 136	Emergency to bring a person from a public place to a place of safety	Transport to safety	Police officer

Common law

Common law is the tradition of law that historically existed in England. It still underpins the English system of law where there is no legal precedent or no codified legislation but a traditional understanding.

In the context of restraint, the common law imperative is that those individuals restraining another individual can account for their actions, which is that they are acting with the authority of the discharge of their professional function.

Principles of good practice

- Explain yourself to the patient or client at the time of restraint.

- Explain yourself to next of kin (if present) at time of restraint.

- Include all involved professionals in the decision-making.

- Encourage a robust critique of the action from your colleagues.

- As soon as is reasonably possible, have a management plan that includes the use of a more structured legal mechanism.

- Have a management or treatment plan.

- Describe in the documentation the events that warrant restraint.

Physical restraint

To restrain somebody physically is an extreme measure and should only be done where there is absolutely no alternative.

Physical restraint must always be undertaken where the human rights of the individual are considered. The risks to leave the individual unrestrained are too great either to themselves or to others.

Physical restraint planning

- Attempt to illicit compliance from patient, explain what is planned if client unable to comply.

- Know the rationale.

- Have a purpose.

- Ensure a team leader is in control.

- Try where possible to have an area where the restraint will be conducted, if this is not possible clear the area of loose objects.

- Assemble sufficient restraint-trained staff.

Physical restraint planning

Team leader to delegate roles of:

- Airway

- Legs one and two

- Arms one and two

- Medication

One person to have sole responsibility for ensuring the airway is at all times clear from obstruction. They should also assume responsibility for protection of the client against head injury.

They should further assume responsibility for ensuring the cervical spine is kept aligned and free of extremes of movement that may cause injury.

One person allocated to each arm.

One person allocated to each leg.

The staff member at each limb is preventing other members of the team from being kicked by immobilising the limb but also trying as much as possible to keep the limb from being put into an unnatural position which could result in injury.

If the purpose of the restraint is to medicate then a team member should have sole responsibility for that function.

Do not

- Hold around the neck.

- Cover face, mouth or nose.

- Hold limbs in a direction abnormal to normal movement.

- Hold by hair or fingers.

Do

- Remain calm.

- Keep control of your team.

- Allow your client the opportunity to access staff therapeutically following this event.

- If you are the team leader allow room for your team to have collective reflection after the event. Critical incident analysis has been shown to be of value in these situations.

- Have an outlet for your own stress and distress, for example clinical supervision.

Rapid tranquillisation

Before tranquillising a client one must ensure every avenue has been explored and the possibility of de-escalation and compliance have been fully explored.

Use an approach that follows a structure and enables clear thinking, planning and conscious decision-making.

Assess the situation: Is there real and present danger?

Consider if the situation is unsafe.

Has the cause for the presented behaviour been considered and managed?

Focus on the patient when making the assessment as this assessment may well be the information which you as a professional have to use to account for your actions in any subsequent review of your management.

Behaviours which might lead to the decision to rapidly tranquillise are:

• Violence to the environment.

• Violence towards others.

• Violence towards self.

• Increasing agitation.

• Threatening and potentially destructive behaviour.

• The making of threats of violence.

• Aggressive gestures.

Rapid tranquillisation should be used in the emergency scenario and the professional in attendance must be convinced that the behaviour in question is consistent and escalating.

Where violence is not a product of organic or mental disorder, then it becomes the domain of the police who should be called.

When planning to proceed with rapid tranquillisation try, where possible, to gain a history and knowledge of current medication and any interactions previously recorded.

Rapid tranquillisation drug regime

This regime is for use when trying to gain control of the acutely disturbed patient

- Assess situation.

- Identify and manage organic causes.

- Attempt to de-escalate by talking down.

> **Always consider any contra indications, potential side effects and interactions with other drugs before administering the following medicines.**
>
> Droperidol 5 to 10mg IM
>
>   and
>
> Lorazepam 2mg IM or IV
>
> *Or*
>
> Haloperidol 2 to 10mg IM or IV
>
>   and
>
> Diazepam 5 to 10mg

Safety and the lone worker

Many healthcare professionals work alone or have to travel alone as an integral part of the job.

Being alone is a vulnerable position both within the context of care and within the context of one's private life.

There are some easily observed behaviours and mechanisms that can reduce risk.

- Always know the patient or client before entering into the caring transaction.
- Read the patient's notes.
- Taking team briefings.
- Be current and aware of changes.

Be conscious and note client behaviour that may indicate a change in the level of risk:

- Violence in speech.
- Expression of violent intent.
- Agitation.
- High energy.
- Smell of alcohol.
- Evidence of drug taking.
- Loss of personal power.
- Need to maintain self-esteem, saving face or peer pressure.

Safety and the lone worker

- Plan interventions.

- Have a clear purpose.

- Consider the physical environment.

- Know where the exit door is and try to avoid allowing your client to come between the door and yourself.

- Plan interventions downstairs if in the client's home.

- Always have the exit in mind.

- If a situation changes act quickly and do not hesitate, leave immediately and return with extra help.

- Avoid stairwells as they are dark, poorly lit and often effectively sound proofed by the heavy fire doors.

Travelling as the lone worker

- If you are in a role that involves travelling to the client's house, this will inevitably involve using a car and using a car in an area that may not be particularly familiar to you. This increases the level of risk.

- Plan your route: Getting lost in an area of deprivation is likely to attract the wrong sort of attention.

- Do not sit in your car writing patient notes or organising equipment. This can give an opportunity for a criminal to get into the passenger side of the car whilst you are distracted.

- When you get into the car immediately lock the doors and then drive away.

- Park your car in a well lit and well observed area.

Useful tip:

If you notice a vehicle, particularly a van, has parked alongside your car; either enter from the opposite side or leave and return later. Many abductions are associated with vans and are carried out whilst the victim is attempting to access their own car.

Travelling as the lone worker

• When walking from your client's house remain aware and cautious.

• Do not use your mobile phone to make calls while in transit. It distracts you and covers up noise from potential attackers.

• Similarly do not use MP3 players or iPods whilst in transit for the same reason.

Risk management behaviour of the lone healthcare worker

- Healthcare workers often consider the needs of others before they consider their own safety. This can lead to their safety being compromised.

- If approached for help consider your safety first.

- Do not give healthcare in an environment that is unsafe.

- While obliged to help, particularly in an emergency, that help may have to be in the form of a call to the emergency service rather than allowing yourself to be put at risk.

- Healthcare workers in the community can be targeted as it is some times assumed that they may be carrying drugs.

Useful tip:

If approached for your medical bag, do not hand your bag to an assailant but rather throw it away from you. The likelihood is that the bag is of more interest and the assailant will go for the bag, giving you the opportunity to run away.

Chapter 16 – Further reading

Chapter 16: Further Reading		
Brewer S	2006	In working order RCN Magazine 43
Source: The Scotsman	2004	Booze-fuelled attacks on medics soar Paramedic UK Scotland
RCN	2005	Working with care : improving working relationships in healthcare RCN publications London
National audit office	2003	A safer place to work: Protecting hospital and ambulance staff from violence and aggression
Mason, T and Chandley, M	1999	Management of Violence and aggression: A Manual for Nurses and Healthcare workers Churchill Livingstone

Chapter 17

Mandatory training: An introduction

In the NHS there have been many new pressures that have put a greater burden on organisations to ensure that their staff are sufficiently trained in the areas that have been considered essential.

This training will vary from organisation to organisation, but will have a principal concern with targeting areas for training that have been shown to have high level of incident of risk and a need for managed quality.

The areas that have been identified for mandatory training typically include:

- Manual Handling.

- Health & Safety.

- Fire safety.

- Infection control.

- Resuscitation (See Chapter 1 and 8).

The following five chapters deal with these issues. Resuscitation has being dealt with in some length in other chapters in this book.

Chapter 18

Moving and Handling

Manual handling is key skill for the healthcare worker. Fundamental to the whole function of nurses, doctors, health support workers or professions allied to medicine is the health and well being of the individual and their capacity to protect their fellow workers from injury in the workplace.

Over 30 per cent of all accidents reported to the Health and Safety Executive are connected with manual handling. Every year 300,000 people are forced to endure the agony of back pain resulting from a manual handling incident. (Unison 2005)

The consequences of back pain are far reaching, affecting not just the work life of the individual but their whole life, as recently reported from a landmark case in South East London where an individual nurse reported that the pain from a back injury sustained at work was so great that she was unable to work in any capacity, unable to pick up her child, and unable to function in any meaningful way.

Back injury from manoeuvring a patient in the workplace can become a life changing and profoundly debilitating injury.

The aspiration of this chapter is to enable the practitioner to move patients and clients in a way that reduces the risk of injury.

The described techniques and information provided are intended to protect the individual practitioner further with an explanation and exploration of:

- Good technique.

- The law.

- Good planning and co-operation at the bed side.

Chapter 18 Contents

Good technique

Position

Position yourself with a good and stable base before attempting a moving and handling manoeuvre.

- Legs apart.

- Knees slightly bent.

- Back straight.

- Close to the patient about to be handled.

Handling

Never risk a handling movement when off balance. Do not rotate or extend spine.

Loads for moving should always be held close to the body.

Never conduct a manual handling manoeuvre in front of the knees or to one side of them.

The vertical 'dead lift' must be avoided.

Communication

Each manoeuvre should have a team leader.

Ensure the patient understands what is about to happen so that they do not move suddenly during the manoeuvre.

Ensure all members of the team are aware of what move is planned.

Achieve a consensus on the command to move on and use a command that has implicit instruction within it. For example:

"Ready, steady slide"

Or

"Ready, steady roll"

The law and manual handling

Manual handling is a function subject to the law, as is any workplace activity that may expose the individual to harm or risk.

Legislation that covers moving and handling is:

- The Health & Safety at Work Act (1974)

- The Management of Health & Safety at Work Regulations (1992)

- Manual Handling Operations Regulations (1992)

MHOR Key principles

- Avoidance

- Assessment

- Reduction of Risk

- Review of Risk

Avoidance

Ensure equipment is available, such as a hoist.

Ensure local culture is one that supports a positive approach to manual handling.

Ensure processes are in place that allow staff rotating within an area to avoid the over exposure of individual team members.

Assessment

Use a structure assessment tool. TILE is covered later in this chapter.

Assess each patient and have an approach available and communicated to your entire team.

Where individual patients are transitory, such as in a theatre environment, it is may be more appropriate to assess individual functions such as moving a patient from bed to theatre table.

Reduction of risk

Use the assessment information to formulate a plan of action that is integral to a plan of care.

Where risk is identified in an environment, use the same structure of assessment to present that risk.

Review of risk

Ensure regular reviews of care and the environment as both can change, warranting changed provision.

TILE

TILE is an acronym that guides the assessment process and ensures a consistent and comprehensive approach.

T =   Task

I =   Individual capability

L =   Load

E =   Environment

Task – note the following in your assessment:

- Holding loads away from the trunk

- Stooping

- Reaching upwards

- Lifting and lowering

- Carrying for long distances

- Strenuous pushing or pulling

- Unpredictability of load

- Repetitive handling recovery periods

- A work rate imposed by a process

- Insufficient rest or recovery periods

Individual capability – note the following in your assessment:

- Hazardous to those with a health problem

- Hazardous to those who are pregnant

- Call for special information or training

- Is movement or posture hindered by clothing or personal protective equipment?

Load – note the following in your assessment:

- Heavy

- Bulky or unwieldy

- Difficult to grasp

- Unstable or unpredictable

- Intrinsically harmful – sharp or hot

Environment – note the following in your assessment:

- Constraints on posture

- Poor floor surfaces

- Variations in levels

- Hot, cold or humid conditions

- Strong air movement

- Poor lighting conditions

Moving and handling – issues for management

Training – ensure a regular process of annual training.

Assessment – good documentation available to all staff.

Equipment and beds – ensure beds and hoists are regularly maintained.

Staffing – adequate staff numbers that increase with workload.

Adequate rest breaks – enable a culture where breaks are routine.

Accident reporting – reporting and auditing accidents enables identification and resolution of problems.

Occupational Health – a good relationship with Occupational Health allows for a proactive model of management of particular health problems.

Vulnerable staff

When responsible for a group of staff, vulnerability of certain groups must be considered and specifically managed:

- Ageing

- History of direct trauma

- Congenital defects

- Pregnancy

- Diabetes and other systemic disorders

- Upper limb disorder

Safe lifting as a consideration within the context of manual handling

In many environments, both within and outside the healthcare environment, there may be times when lifting is expected.

This would include lifting of equipment and patients. The diagram below shows the safe weight to lift relative to the position of the bearer's body.

It always better to avoid lifting. Even when the weights are as small as this, there remains a degree of risk.

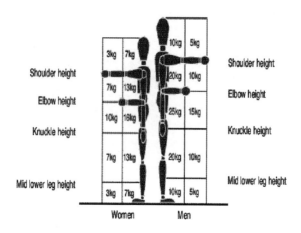

Manual handling equipment: The hoist

Generic principles of the hoist

There are many hoists available and most will have common features. Knowledge of these common features can help the practitioner to use these aids in a safe way.

Hoists are mechanical equipment and will have features that relate to safe use of electrical and mechanical equipment.

Weight limit

Ensure your hoist has the correct weight tolerance; typically this is between 140 and 170kg.

The very obese will need specialist equipment.

Maintenance

All equipment should be regularly maintained, at least yearly. The maintenance record should be displayed on the hoist.

Ensure there are fully charged batteries before using the hoist. In the event of a failure mid manoeuvre, the hoist will often have a fail-safe backup. This provides access to a small reserve of power to help the lowering of a patient to a safe position.

The hoist slings

Ensure that the sling is the correct sling for this hoist.

The sling will come in different sizes that are denoted either by a colour coding, usually on the border of the sling or noted on the tab at the back.

Using the hoist

When using the hoist ensure there is a team leader who has control of this equipment. This will ensure the management of the team and the safe use of the equipment.

Explain to the patient and the rest of the team what is planned.

Position the sling by either rolling the patient on to the sling if in the lying position, or by sliding the sling into place if in the sitting position.

Deploying the hoist

- Lift the hoist arm up and out of the way.

- Separate hoist legs to ensure proximity to the patient and a wide base from which to lift the patient.

Lower the hoist arm

- Attach the sling ensuring it is correctly attached. Some hoists will have the bottom tabs deployed to the outside of the patient's legs, whilst other sling tabs are deployed in-between the patient's legs.

- **Caution**: If the sling is wrongly deployed there is a possibility of abducting the patients legs as they are lifted which can make the patient feel particularly vulnerable especially if they are in a state of undress.

- A further concern is that abduction of the legs in this fashion of a patient with a recent hip replacement can cause displacement of the hip prosthesis.

Preparing to lift with the hoist

- Once the patient is in position, explain again what is to happen as this is a potentially frightening experience for them.

- Immediately before the lift commences, the team leader should ensure that the patient's arms are within the sling.

If the arms are outside the sling and holding on to adjacent structures, there is the possibility of disruption to the dynamic between the swinging loads of the patient in the sling and the supporting structure of the hoist arm. This can result in the patient swinging wildly and banging their head on the hoist arm.

No equipment, such as catheters, drains, intravenous infusion lines should be attached and fixed outside of the sling. There is a risk that when the hoist is in motion the tension through this equipment may cause traumatic removal and injury.

When lifting the patient in the hoist leave the brakes off: This ensures that as the patient moves, the hoist can adjust its base in relation to load relative to the changing centre of gravity that the moving patient represents.

Moving and handling equipment: Slide sheets

Slide sheets are a very effective aid in manual handling and are inexpensive to purchase compared to equipment such as hoists.

Slide sheets work by reducing friction and therefore the effort needed to move a patient.

They are designed to slide over another surface with the same friction lowering properties, that is, to slide over another slide sheet. If the sheet is designed in a circular or tubular form then they slide across its other surface in motion that could approximate a roll.

Slide sheets are not designed to slide across bed sheets as this will reduce their efficiency.

Preparing the patient

- With the lying patient, position them into the angel position, that is, flat on the back with arms crossed across the chest.

- From this position, bend the leg so that the knee points upwards.

Position two carers to the side of the patient then identify the three anchor points of hip, knee and shoulder.

- The carers can place their hands on to all three anchor points, crossing arms at the hip.

- From this position, the patient is rolled on the command "Ready, Steady, Roll."

- The rolled up slide sheet can now be positioned under the patient and then the manoeuvre can be repeated in the opposite direction.

- Once the slide sheet is positioned under the patient, it is important to ensure that the entire body of the patient is within the scope of the slide sheet as small areas such as the feet outside the slide sheet can cause dramatic loss of efficiency and add to the carer's workload.

- When moving the patient on the slide sheet carers should be positioned on either side of the patient and should coordinate the manoeuvre on the command "Ready, Steady, Slide."

Slide sheets with PAT slides

When slide sheets are used with the PAT slide, they are deployed in the same way as previously described. However there are further considerations that should be observed in these instances:

- Slide sheets should always be used in conjunction with the PAT slide.

- Never use a bed sheet with the PAT slide. This is not licensed to be used in this way and if there is a problem such as the sheet tearing the patient could be injured. The liability would be with the carer or nurse rather than the employing authority.

- PAT slides are most often used to transfer a patient from bed to bed or trolley to bed. In this situation, always use extensions to the slide sheet in order to avoid stretching to reach the patient and the common and unsafe practice of getting on to the bed and sliding the patient towards yourself.

Chapter 18 – Further reading

Chapter 18: Further Reading		
Health & Safety Executive	1999	Management of health & safety at work regulations approved code of practice Stationery office London
Health & Safety Executive	2003	Understanding ergonomics at work Stationery office London
National Back Exchange	2001	Manual handling training guidelines Column 13(3), 12-13
Royal College of Nursing	2000	Manual handling training guidance: Competencies for manual handling RCN London
Health & Safety executive	2004	Are you making the best of lifting and handling aids HSE Books Suffolk
HSE Books	2004	The Manual Handling Operations Regulations 1992 Guidance on Regulations

General Health and Safety

Health and Safety is the responsibility of both the employer and the employee. This mandatory obligation is stated within the Health and Safety at Work Act 1974.

Employers have a duty to maintain health and safety standards and have to take reasonable steps to ensure the health, safety and welfare of their employees at work.

Chapter 19 Contents

Health & Safety obligations

As an employee, you have a duty to take reasonable care of your own and other's health and safety.

Employees must read and be familiar with:

- Fire policy.

- Health & Safety manual.

- Infection control policy and procedure.

Risk Assessment:

- Employers must conduct regular risk assessments in the areas of work

- In the year 2004/05, the Health and Safety Executive reported that in the UK, 220 workers and 361 members of the public were killed, and 363,000 people suffered an injury due to accidents at work.

- All incidents and near misses need to be reported.

Working environment, the employer's obligations

The employer must provide basic facilities to make the work place safe and healthy:

- Enough space to work.

- Floors should be kept clean and in good repair.

- Stairways fitted with guard rails, floor openings must be covered and guarded.

- Fire escapes kept clear and well marked.

- Sufficient toilet accommodation, drinking water and hand washing facilities must be available.

- Comfortable working temperature and ventilation.

- Good standard of lighting.

Health & Safety: Hazardous substances at work

- 1,000 new chemicals are developed every year.

- All persons using chemicals must ensure that they are used, handled and stored correctly.

- Many toxic and harmful chemicals are used in hospitals for cleaning and disinfection.

Regulated by the Control of Substances Hazardous to Health (1988)

Health & Safety: RIDDOR

RIDDOR: Reporting of Injuries, Diseases and Dangerous Occurrences Regulations 1995

- Reporting accidents and ill health at work is a legal requirement.

RIDDOR reporting:

- Death or major injury

- Three day injury

- Disease

- Dangerous occurrence

Ensure a good record is kept of any such occurrence. This should tie in with the incident reporting form in the workplace.

Health & Safety: Equipment

Equipment must be properly maintained and placed away safely after use.

There is a precedent of a Trust being successfully sued for breech of Health & Safety law in the instance of poorly stored and infected sharps causing injury to an unauthorised intruder. See Chapter 4 – Dealing with needlestick injury.

Health & Safety: Fire safety

Between 900 and 1,000 people each year die in fires. Around 30 of these are as a result of fires in the work place.

Main causes:

- Arson

- Smoking

- Electrical fires

Employees are obliged to know where fire doors and escape routes are located.

Employers must have a fire policy which all employees must read.

Health & Safety: Violence and aggression

Violence and aggression towards healthcare workers is on the increase. We are all at risk, no matter where we work.

All cases of violence or aggression must be reported.

Escape routes – always have a door or escape route behind you, and be able to back away.

Never get trapped in a cubicle with an aggressor

Avoid confrontation and arguments, trust gut instinct. See Chapter 16.

Health & Safety: Occupational Health

The Occupational Health Department has a vital function in maintaining the well being of staff. The department also responds to issues of health and risk that have an impact on the individual employee in the workplace.

The chronology of care provided by Occupational Health Departments begins with the pre-employment interview, which is both surveillance and proactive, providing:

• Advice and guidance.

• Vaccinations, for example Hepatitis B.

Subsequently, Occupational Health manage issues that can arise, including:

• Work related injury or stress.

• Latex allergy.

• Needlestick injury.

• Confidential advice on any health problem.

Chapter 19 – Further reading

Chapter 19: Further Reading

Health & Safety Executive	1999	Management of health & safety at work regulations approved code of practice Stationery office London
Health & Safety Executive	2003	Understanding ergonomics at work Stationery office London
National Back Exchange	2001	Manual handling training guidelines Column 13(3), 12-13
Royal College of Nursing	2000	Manual handling training guidance: Competencies for manual handling RCN London
Health & Safety executive	2004	Are you making the best of lifting and handling aids HSE Books Suffolk
HSE Books	2004	The Manual Handling Operations Regulations 1992 Guidance on Regulations

Chapter 20

Fire Safety

A fundamental responsibility of all staff in the workplace is the vigilant observance of fire safety. This is of particular significance where the population in a healthcare environment can have impaired mobility due to the nature of their illness.

A further consideration for the healthcare profession is the duty of care that they have in relation to their patients. This puts extra onus on the professional's proactive observance of good conduct in relation to fire but also in good management in the instance of fire.

Chapter 20 Contents

Fire Safety: Legislation

The legislation which currently governs conduct with fire safety is:

• Fire Precautions Act 1971

• Fire Precautions (Workplace) Regulations 1997

The above legislation is scheduled to be withdrawn when the new Regulatory Reform (Fire Safety) Order becomes law.

Originally due in April 2006, this legislation has been delayed and is not likely to be implemented before October 2006.

Fire Safety

A compliant and safe environment should have a strategy in place that encompasses the following.

Provision of safety guidelines and regulations

- Fire procedure

- Evacuation procedure

Building provision

- Fire exits

- Fire doors to enable containment of fire

Hazards

- Hazards should be identified in the work place and special provision made

- Integral to other procedures should be recognition of the risk of fire

For example, the use of oxygen in the instance of defibrillation.

Fire-fighting equipment

Integral to the fabric of the building should be the provision of, and access to, water supply for the Fire Service.

Fire Safety: Training

Hospitals and other healthcare environments are obliged to provide training that enables a safe environment which will include:

- Training in assessment of response to fire.

- Call for help with 999 call and *break glass*, and/or emergency call to the switchboard.

- How to use a fire extinguisher.

- Knowledge of exit routes.

- Fire doors, their purpose in preventing the spread of fire and their barrier function in the instance of lateral evacuation.

- Local assembly points.

- The appointment and specialist training of a local fire marshal.

- Location of the fire extinguisher.

- Understanding of evacuation procedure.

Fire Safety: Fire Extinguishers

The requirements of the new standard, BS EN 3, are that all fire extinguishers are coloured RED, although BS 7863 allows the UK to have 3% to 5% (usually the label) of the extinguisher body colour coded in accordance with the 'old' system.

Extinguisher	Best for:	Caution
Water	Carboniferous, wood, cloth, paper, coal etc. Fires involving solids	Do not use on burning fat or oil on electrical appliances
Dry Powder	Wood, cloth, paper, plastics, coal etc. Fires involving solids. Liquids such as grease, fats, oil, paint, petrol etc.	Safe on live electrical. Do not use on chip or fat pan fires.

Extinguisher	Best for:	Caution
 CO_2 **Carbon Dioxide**	Liquids such as grease, fats, oil paint, petrol etc.	Do not use on chip or fat pan fires. CO2 can be harmful so ventilate the area as soon as the fire has been confirmed as extinguished.
 Foam	Petrol and volatile liquids. Ideal for multi-risk usage.	Do not use on electrical and chip pan fires as the foam is water based.
 Fire Blanket	Fires involving solids and liquids. Particularly good for small fires in clothing and for chip and fat pan fires **provided the blanket completely covers the fire**.	If the blanket does not completely cover the fire, it will not be able to extinguish the fire. Do not remove the blanket until it is cool

Fire Safety: Fire Marshals

The fire marshal is an important provision in the management of fire safety in that at a time of extremis, there needs to be a clear direction and no delay.

The marshal has the following responsibilities:

- To be identifiable by wearing the fire marshal tabard.

- Provide information and a point of contact.

- Roll call: Ensure all staff and patients are accounted for.

- Where the fire marshal is also operational, they may also have extended responsibilities for liaison and evacuation.

Chapter 20 – Further reading

Chapter 20: Further Reading		
Health & Safety Executive	1999	Management of Health & Safety at work regulations approved code of practice Stationery office London
Health & Safety Executive	2003	Understanding ergonomics at work Stationery office London
National Back Exchange	2001	Manual handling training guidelines Column 13(3), 12-13
Royal College of Nursing	2000	Manual handling training guidance: Competencies for manual handling RCN London
Health & Safety Executive	2004	Are you making the best of lifting and handling aids HSE Books Suffolk
HSE Books	2004	The Manual Handling Operations Regulations 1992 Guidance on Regulations

Chapter 21

Infection control

Infection control is a key concern for any professional involved with patients that are subject to our duty of care. They can expect precautions are taken to protect them from the problems associated with acquired infection.

Any contact with the healthcare environment and care professionals should a have a positive outcome for the individual and not result in a worsening of their circumstances.

Chapter 21 Contents

Universal precautions

Universal precautions is an approach to the unknown risk presented by the handling of body products and provides a safe system for the healthcare professional.

This is done while maintaining a consistent approach to the patient in order that confidential information of infection is not identified by the behaviour of the healthcare professional.

Universal precautions is a method of care delivery that recognises all body products from all patients constitute a risk, and therefore stipulate the use of a barrier between healthcare professionals and body products.

Caution should therefore be taken with all blood and body products.

The following is a list of the less common body products that still constitute a risk

Blood and bloody fluids and other body substances

- Blood and wound excaudate
- Faeces
- Urine
- Saliva
- Breast milk
- Semen
- Vaginal secretions
- Cerebral spinal fluid
- Synovial fluid
- Pleural fluid
- Peritoneal fluid
- Pericardial fluid
- Amniotic fluid
- Unfixed organs and tissue

The most effective barrier is the disposable glove.

Caution: there is a high and growing instance of allergy in response to latex and it is prudent to keep non-latex gloves in all clinical environments for staff that have been sensitised.

The spread of infection

The spread of infection is often referred to as the chain of infection because of the interlinked sequence of events. These are:

- A causal agent – the organism responsible.

- A reservoir – hospital equipment.

- A portal of entry – where the skin integrity is compromised, for example at the site of an infusion.

- A mode of transmission – from the hand of the attendant carer.

- A portal of exit – the point of contact.

Breaking this chain of events at any point will result in an effective reduction of the incidence of infection.

Hospital acquired infection (HAI)

There are thought to be approximately one million people affected by hospital acquired infection (HAI) at any one time in the UK. This provides a very compelling mandate for a robust policy of infection control.

The hospital population of patients are prone to acquired infection due to:

- Invasive procedures.

- Patient vulnerability due to underlying illness.

- Prolonged hospital stays which is effectively prolonged exposure to other organisms resident in that environment.

Bacteria and the spread of infection

There are always micro-organisms resident on the skin of the hands which can be classified into two broadly defined types which behave differently and have different implications for our approach to infection control. These two groups are resident and transient.

Resident	Transient
Deep seated.	Superficial.
Difficult to remove.	Transfer with ease.
Part of body's natural defence.	An important source of cross infection.
Associated with infection following surgery.	Easily removed with good hand washing.

Good hand washing removes both resident and transient, but particular effort is needed to remove the deep seated resident bacteria such as in the preparation for surgery.

Hand washing

Hands should be washed in:

- Soap and water

- Chlorhexidine Gluconate

- Providine iodine

- Triclosan

1. Palm to palm

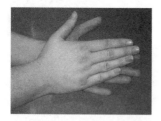

2. Right palm over left dorsum, and left palm over right dorsum.

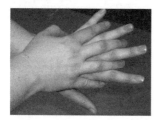

3. Palm to palm, fingers interlaced.

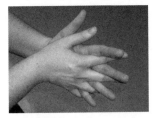

4. Backs of fingers to opposing palms with fingers interlocked.

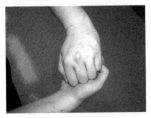

5. Rotational rubbing of right thumb clasped in left palm and vice versa.

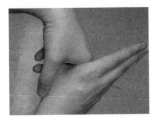

6. Rotational rubbing, clasped in left palm and vice versa backwards and forwards with clasped of right hand in left palm and vice versa.

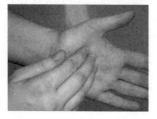

Methacillin resistant staphylococcal aureus (MRSA)

MRSA is the identified organism in 20% of all staphylococcal aureus cultures in the UK. Its incidence seems to be growing in number and it is increasingly responsible for major illness.

Managing MRSA is a significant responsibility of all healthcare workers in every environment.

Proactive management:

- Consider every source contaminated

- Isolate all new admissions until proven negative of MRSA carriage

- Pre-admission screening

- If at all possible manage patients away from healthcare environment if known positive

- Have robust process of screening

Three consecutive negative screens

Each swab taken on different days

Swabs to be from more than one site on each screening

When MRSA has been identified in an environment:

- Identify the source

- Isolate with barrier nursing

- Treat infected patients and staff

- Terminal clean

- Close ward or hospital.

Needlestick injury

- Make the wound bleed under cold tap

- Report immediately to the Accident and Emergency department

- Risk assessment to consider need for Post-Exposure Prophylaxis (PEP)

- Report to senior operational manager

- Occupational health

- Draw blood from the donor to identify the level of risk if the HIV status is unknown, this will need the consent of the donor patient.

See Chapter 4.

Chapter 21 – Further reading

Chapter 21: Further Reading

Dietze B, Rath A, Wendt C & Martiny	2001	Survival of MRSA on sterile goods packaging Journal of hospital infection 49(4) 3255-261
Department of Health	2001	Standard principles for preventing hospital acquired infection Journal of hospital infection 47(Supp), S21-37
Menon K V, Whiteley P, Burden RB, Galland B	1999	Surgical patients with methicillin resistance staphylococcus aureus infection: an analysis of outcome using P-POSSUM J.R.College Surgery. (44) 161-3
Wilson, J	2001	Infection Control in Clinical Practice Bailliere Tindall
Horton, R, Parker, L	2002	Informed Infection Control Practice Churchill Livingstone

Chapter 22

Basic life support

Basic life support training is mandatory for all healthcare workers and, in many organisations, for non-healthcare staff working in the healthcare environment such as reception staff in doctors' surgeries.

The resuscitation algorithm is shown on the next page, for information in greater depth see Chapters 1 and Chapter 6.

Adult Basic Life Support

Resuscitation Council (UK) 2005

Adult Basic Life Support

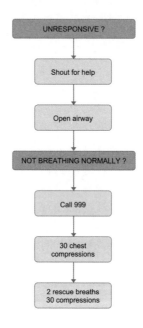

Chapter 23

The use of a reflective diary

A defining purpose underpinning the writing of this book was a concern for the professional in new areas of practice. Whether these are new enhancements to the clinical function like diagnostics and prescription, or new management challenges such as the nurse leading the Hospital at Night team.

Within this chapter, that concern is brought in to greater focus with a description of a structure and process that may be of value for the professional in the process of new skill acquisition and consolidation of those skills.

The reflective journal is intended as an aid to enable the practitioner to record new encounters and reconcile those with prior knowledge, or reconcile them with the literary resource of this book and with literature and knowledge further a field.

It is also envisaged that the record generated by the practitioner using this reflective journal, when coupled with further literature, could become the bedrock of evidenced learning from which further learning and development goals could be planned.

A further strength of a reflective diary is that it encourages the practitioner to reflection which can be achieved without or indeed within a clinical supervisory relationship.

A benefit of this reflective infrastructure is that it can add a level of supportive value, in that it can enable a process of catharsis and closure when a traumatic or difficult event is recorded in a written format.

Chapter 23 Contents

The use of a reflective diary

It is envisaged that this record could indeed become a tool to identify learning needs and when those learning needs have been met, which could further be used as an evidential source for transition through a gateway as described in the knowledge and skills framework structure.

The format of the diary is as follows:

1.0   Account experience

2.0   Contemporaneous reflection

3.0   Relevant data source

4.0   New insights and new learning

Example reflective diary

Date	Account experience
	On the night of the 23rd I was called to Mary Ward and I found a very confused and agitated man who was running around the ward threatening violence and throwing things to the floor.

On the night of the 23rd I was called to Mary Ward and I found a very confused and agitated man who was running around the ward threatening violence and throwing things to the floor.

The patient was a de-toxing alcoholic who had not been given any sedation since admission some 48 hours previously.

I quickly assessed the situation and felt that the patients' violence was a source of risk to both staff and patients.

There was no security or doctors in attendance.

Actions taken:

I emergency called the security team

The medical SHO was then called to the ward

When all members of the team were in place we attempted to de-escalate the situation and offered the patient some oral haloperidol which was refused. The patient was becoming increasingly agitated and verbalising violent intent towards the staff present.

A decision was made to restrain the patient and give the drug intra muscularly

The process of restraint was co-ordinated by myself with each of the patients limbs allocated to a security team member. Responsibility for maintaining airway and cervical spine safety given to the ward nurse in attendance. The medication was given successfully.

Contemporaneous reflection *(To be undertaken as soon as possible at the time or soon after the event)*

When I went to the ward initially I felt very anxious and a little frightened, I felt this man was going to attack someone and there did not seem to be a way of stopping him or containing the situation.

I was made anxious by the fact that everybody was looking to me for management of the situation and I wasn't sure what to do.

After the situation was managed I felt uncomfortable about the fact that we held somebody down against their will and I was anxious that we may have contravened his human rights.

Relevant data source

I discussed this with my colleagues

I looked at the hospital issued information about legal mechanisms for restraint

I also looked at the rapid tranquillisation policy

I explored the internet for information on the human rights act.

New insights and new learning

Following on from this experience and my subsequent resourced reflection I felt that the best way to manage this situation would have been pro actively with medication prescribed on admission as per detoxification protocol.

Subsequently I will always ensure that admitted patients with this problem have had this addressed.

My concerns about the human rights were well founded and it would seem that this practice is untested in terms of The Human Rights Act, although I think the management of this situation in this way is not uncommon and the legal mechanism used is described as

"Common law" (I think I will read more on this subject as it seems at times unclear)

I was happy with the way that the restraint was managed in that we were particularly effective and acted in a way to protect the patient, taking particular care of the airway and the cervical spine.

Date	Account experience
	Contemporaneous reflection
	Relevant data source
	New insights and new learning

Chapter 23 – Further reading

Chapter 23: Further Reading		
Palmer A, Burns S, Bulman C	1994	Reflective practice in nursing: The growth of the professional practitioner London Blackwell
Powell J H	1989	The reflective practitioner in nursing Journal of advanced nursing 14, 824-832
Palmer A, Burns S, Bulman C	1994	Reflective practice in nursing: The growth of the professional practitioner London Blackwell
Powell J H	1989	The reflective practitioner in nursing Journal of advanced nursing 14, 824-832
Heath H B M (Ed)	2002	Foundations in nursing theory and practice London Mosby
Joshua A King T (Eds)	1996	Guy's hospital nursing drug reference London Mosby
O'Conner N	2006	Prescription for change RCN Magazine 21-25

Chapter 23: Further Reading

Dougherty L, Lister S (Eds)	2004	The Royal Marsden Hospital manual of clinical nursing practice 6th Edition London Blackwell

Index